Practical Intervention for Early Childhood Stammering

Palin PCI Approach

Practical Intervention for Early Childhood Stammering

Palin PCI Approach

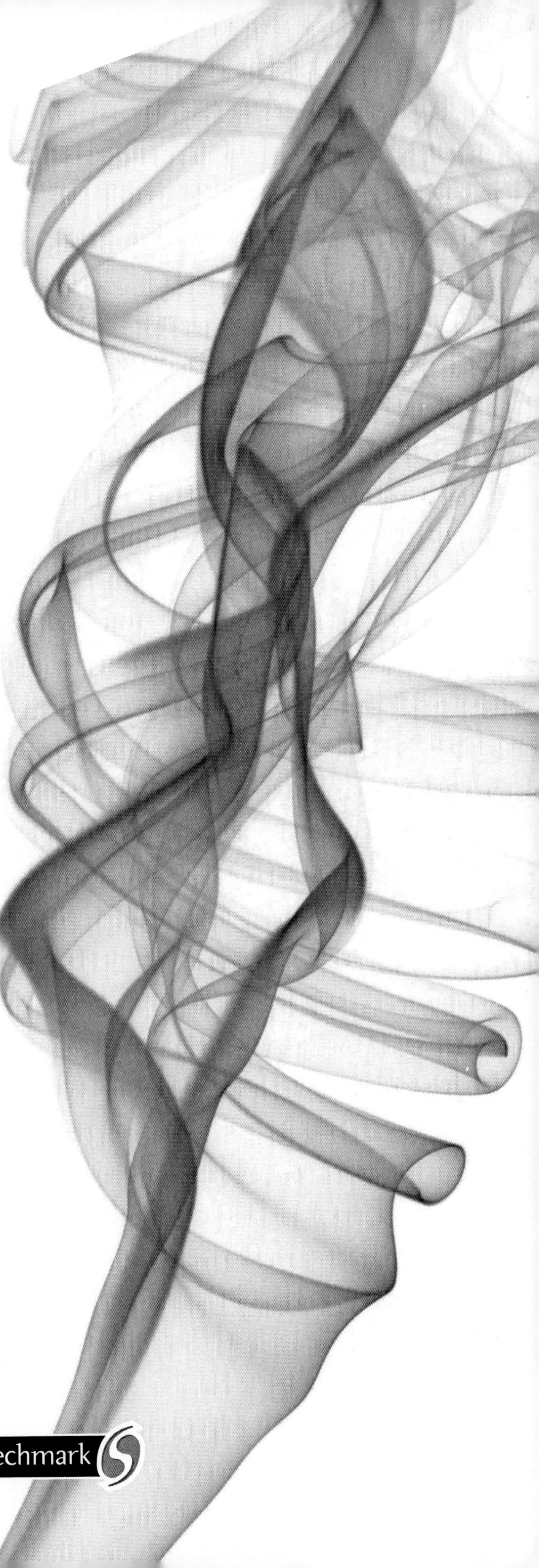

Elaine Kelman &
Alison Nicholas

Speechmark

First published in 2008 by
Speechmark Publishing Ltd, Sunningdale House, 43 Caldecotte Lake Drive, Milton Keynes MK7 8LF, United Kingdom
Tel: +44 (0)1908 277177 Fax: +44 (0)1908 278297
www.speechmark.net

Reprinted 2011 (twice), 2013 (twice)

002-5433/Printed in the United Kingdom by CMP (uk) Ltd.

British Library Cataloguing in Publication Data

Kelman, Elaine
Practical intervention for early childhood stammering : Palin PCI approach
1. Stuttering in children – Treatment
I. Title II. Nicholas, Alison
618.9'2855406

ISBN 978 0 86388 667 6

To Diana de Grunwald, who has always been at the heart of the Michael Palin Centre – providing gracious support to the families and strength and encouragement to all her colleagues. We all owe her so much.

Contents

List of Figures

Foreword

'It is the province of knowledge to speak, and it is the privilege of wisdom to listen.'

Oliver Wendell Holmes

Some approach childhood stuttering with mainly child-related strategies while others approach it with mainly family-related strategies. It would seem that the former place the onus on nature while the latter consider nurture to be the main causal contributor to developmental stuttering. Fortunately, there is no such categorical, black or white thinking anywhere in this book by Elaine Kelman and Alison Nicholas. These authors recognise, as it were, that the child swims in a communicative sea provided by the family but that some children, right from the beginning, are better communicative swimmers than others, regardless of how stormy the sea may be.

Starting from a base of clearly explicated theory, involving a multifactorial model of stuttering, the authors lay out what are for them some of the more important risk factors for beginning as well as continuing to stutter. While it will be some time before we fully appreciate the relative value of these various risk factors for predicting continuance of childhood stuttering, the authors take a reasoned, even-handed approach that clinicians will benefit from considering. The two authors have written the thin line between the nature and nurture divide.

By so doing, these authors show that we can make further progress in the treatment of childhood stuttering if we ground our empirically-derived clinical method in relevant theory and provide evidential motivation for that which we do clinically. Indeed, the authors provide evidence for their approach. And while one may argue about their (or anyone else's) evidence, they provide it for us to see and consider. Indeed, while critics of X, Y or Z treatments frequently ask 'what's the evidence?' seldom do they ask, 'who decides?' and/or 'who decides what the evidence should be?' Rather, implicit in these critics' comments is the notion that they are the self-appointed thumbs-up/thumbs-down arbitrators of what treatments live or die in the free marketplace of therapeutic approaches from which we all must carefully and thoughtfully select. However, these two authors take no such inflexible stand and avoid such polemics as they explicate their approach, the motivation as well as evidence for it. Recognising that nothing works for everybody – not penicillin, not aspirin, not back surgery – the authors provide a logical progression of 'steps,' from assessment to treatment, but do so without claiming nor falling into the one-size-fits-all trap too often seen with the treatment of childhood stuttering.

Throughout the text one thing is clear: these authors have established their clinical *ethos* built on years of clinical experience. What they do with this book is to tie their clinical ethos ever closer together with modern-day research/ theoretical *logos* and to provide – by their excellent case studies – humanistic *pathos* to create a cohesive, motivated approach to the management of childhood stuttering.

Kelman and Nicholas make clear the importance of *interaction* between the child and his environment when trying to assess and treat children who stutter. Consistently recognising the bi-directionality of this interaction, these two authors, from the first chapter to the last, weave a sturdy net of ideas and approaches that attempts to capture salient aspects of the child, his environment and interactions between the two.

Given the capturing powers of their observational net, the authors' approach is quite *flexible* in that once they establish the child's concerns through their assessment, they are able to attend to the special needs of the individual child and the child's family whilst being able to deal with that which is common between this child and all others. Such flexibility also comes from the fact that few relevant considerations appear to be overlooked and the fact that the authors provide a rationale for assessing the many subtle but significant variables that may affect the child's speech fluency, for example, disturbances to the equilibrium of the family due to problems of a sibling.

Making explicit one of the more thorough diagnostic approaches to be found in the entire literature pertaining to childhood stuttering, the authors provide a *continuity* of approach that ties together the whole of their clinical practice. For example, from the very beginning, these authors attempt to ground treatment in assessment, much as they attempt to ground practice in theory. This approach leads to a continuity of thought and practice that serves to make their approach logical as well as defendable, to both consumers and professionals alike.

This book is written throughout in a straightforward manner and the practising clinician should find it easy to grasp the authors' approach and ideas. Liberally supported throughout with clinical observations and case studies, the book seldom strays from its central topic – assessment and treatment of childhood stuttering – and this focus should provide a strong incentive to anyone interested in learning more about the assessment and treatment of childhood stuttering.

Reading this book often reminds one of looking through an observation window at master clinicians plying their trade. We not only read about the art and science of their approach, but what these clinicians believe they are doing, when and why. Thus, although it is not possible for us to actually observe these authors providing clinical services or interview them afterwards about the same, this book gives us a somewhat similar experience. Enjoy. I think you will!

Edward Gage Conture
Vanderbilt University
Nashville, TN
USA

Acknowledgements

This book is long overdue. We started to write it some time ago, and, in the process, began to reflect on our work and gradually adapt and revise it to its current form: Palin PCI.

The book represents a team effort, originally inspired by Lena Rustin, but then developed into a coherent therapy package by Willie Botterill. We would like to acknowledge the input provided by all our colleagues at the Michael Palin Centre, especially Ali Biggart, Jane Fry and Sharon Millard. A special thank you to Sharon, who has kept us on our research toes.

Frances Cook has been a source of unfailing wisdom, patience and support, guiding us with clarity and insight through our many drafts.

Of course, our inspiration has come from the many children and their families whom we have worked with over the years. They have taught us so much.

We would also like to thank the following for their generous support:

- Trustees of the Association for Research into Stammering in Childhood
- Islington Primary Care Trust
- The Wessex Youth Trust.

We are indebted to Michael Palin for all he does for us and for allowing us to use his name.

Finally, we would like to thank our husbands and families for their patience, tolerance and encouragement.

Elaine Kelman and Alison Nicholas

1

Introduction

Young children who stammer (CWS) usually present in a generalist clinic. We know from research and experience that early intervention is effective (Jones *et al*, 2005; Millard *et al*, 2008). However, stammering is not a simple problem to understand or to treat, and research has also shown us that many speech & language therapists (SLTs) are anxious about treating CWS (Crichton-Smith *et al*, 2003). This book has been written to give SLTs guidance and the confidence to assess and treat young children referred to them because of concerns about their fluency.

Over many years the Michael Palin Centre for Stammering Children (MPC) has provided training to hundreds of therapists, giving them the skills they need to treat young children effectively. We know that accessing training is sometimes difficult, so this book is intended to help more therapists to provide early intervention. However, a book cannot replace a training course, where therapists will learn, through watching videos and doing practical exercises, the methods and skills demonstrated. We recommend that learning from this book is enhanced through initially working alongside another therapist where possible.

Our most recent book on the treatment of early childhood stammering was published in 1996 (Rustin *et al*, 1996), and since then our philosophy and methods have evolved significantly. We view the child who stammers as having abilities and vulnerabilities that have contributed to the stammering problem. We also recognise that parents are often instinctively managing their child's stammer in helpful ways and we aim to work with them to identify and build on the knowledge they already have.

In this first chapter we present our theoretical framework, which helps to identify and understand the factors that contribute to the onset, development and persistence of stammering. We provide research and clinical evidence for this framework.

This is followed by a description of how the Palin Parent–Child Interaction therapy (Palin PCI) approach evolved as a method of treating early childhood stammering, and we provide research and clinical evidence for its components and its methods. We outline our recent research, which demonstrates the efficacy of Palin PCI, in order to assure therapists and managers that this approach forms evidence-based practice.

We then outline alternative care pathways for early stammering, based on evidence about a child's level of vulnerability to persistence. The 'Advice and Monitoring' care pathway is designed for a child who is likely to recover, and the 'Full Assessment and Palin PCI' care pathway is for the child who is likely to persist in stammering.

In Chapter 4 we describe the assessment and case history protocols that identify the child's abilities and vulnerabilities, as well as any other factors which may be contributing to his stammer. We demonstrate how this information may then be used to understand each child's stammering, the appropriate therapy components, and how to present this in a 'formulation' for the parents. All assessment forms, charts and other resources are included on the accompanying CD-ROM for printing and copying as required.

In Chapters 6 and 7 we present the Palin PCI approach, showing how interaction and family strategies are integrated to support the child's fluency. The sequence and techniques are described in detail, and we provide handouts that may be given to parents as an added resource. Strategies for working directly on the child's fluency are included, together with guidance on other important issues such as working with preschool and school staff. We have included troubleshooting sections which are based on questions typically asked by therapists during our training courses.

Palin PCI is highly accessible to SLTs because it taps into and develops the many skills they are already using in managing the rest of their caseload. They can then apply Palin PCI principles and methods to other speech and language difficulties, and thus develop their clinical skills more widely (Cummins & Hulme, 1997).

We illustrate the Palin PCI approach with three case studies based on the children and families we have worked with. We have also included observations made by parents, in order to provide some real-life user feedback.

In line with the usual conventions, we have used 'he' when referring to the child, and 'she' when referring to the therapist.

We believe that Palin PCI is a straightforward and logical way to treat children who stammer. It is also an interesting and fun way of working with families.

We hope you will agree!

What is stammering?

Stammering occurs in all parts of the world, across all cultures, religions and socio-economic groups. It is a complex problem that may be referred to as 'stammering', 'stuttering' or 'dysfluency'.

Although the quantity and type of stammering differs for each individual, the following features are more usual.

- Repetition of whole words, for example *'and, and, and then I left'*.
- Repetition of single syllables, for example *'c-c-come h-h-here'*.
- Prolonging of sounds, for example *'sssssssometimes I go out'*.
- Blocking of sounds, where the mouth is in position, but no sound comes out.
- Facial tension in the muscles around the eyes, nose, lips or neck.
- Extra body movements may occur as the child attempts to 'push' the word out, for example stamping his feet, shifting body position or tapping with his fingers.
- The breathing pattern may be disrupted, for example the child may hold his breath while speaking or take an exaggerated breath before speaking.

Sometimes the child adopts strategies to try and minimise or hide the problem, for example:

- Avoiding or changing words: the child may say *'I've forgotten what I was going to say'* or may switch to another word when he begins to stammer, for example, *'I played with my br- br- br...my sister on Saturday'*.
- Avoiding certain situations: for instance, not contributing during 'circle time' at preschool or not putting his hand up to answer a question at school.

Some children become so adept at hiding their problem in this manner that they may appear fluent, or they may just become very quiet.

Onset of stammering

Most stammering begins in early childhood, usually appearing between the age of two and four years, coinciding with a period of rapid expansion of speech and language skills (Yairi & Ambrose, 2005). The onset of stammering is typically gradual, but in cases where the onset was reported to be sudden, Yairi and Ambrose (1992a) found that the stammering was more likely to be severe.

Who is affected?

Around the time when it first emerges, the ratio of boys to girls affected by stammering is equal (Kloth *et al*, 1999; Yairi, 1983). However, by the time children start at school, the ratio is three boys to every one girl, and by the age of 10 years it is 5:1 or 6:1. (Bloodstein & Bernstein Ratner, 2007).

The prevalence of stammering (how many people currently stammer) in the general population is approximately one per cent (Bloodstein & Bernstein Ratner, 2007). The incidence rate (how many people have stammered at some time in their lives) is approximately four to five per cent, which reflects the large proportion of children who recover spontaneously (Andrews *et al*, 1983; Yairi & Ambrose 2005).

Individuality and variability

One common feature of early stammering is its apparent unpredictability and variability. A child's stammer may vary from day to day and from one situation to another, and is influenced by a number of different factors, including the child's language (Weiss & Zebrowski, 2000), the context in which he is speaking (Yaruss, 1997), the interaction style of the person he is talking to (Guitar *et al*, 1992: Guitar & Marchinkoski, 2001), as well as how the child is feeling at the time. Phases of stammering are often interspersed by fluent periods, which may last for weeks, and it is often difficult to identify any reasons for these fluctuations.

Why do some children stammer?

The simple answer to this question is that we do not know. For decades researchers have been trying to find out why people stammer and, to date, no single factor can account for its development. People who stammer are heterogeneous individuals and research findings are conflicting. Group results do not necessarily reflect the performance of the individuals involved. Many studies have only included a small number of subjects and their results cannot be generalised to the stammering population as a whole. Consequently, interpretation of research findings is a challenge.

There is general consensus among experts that many factors are influential in both the onset and the development of stammering. Many of these are reported in the research literature, while others have arisen from clinical expertise (see Conture, 2001; Guitar, 2006; Riley & Riley, 1979; Rustin *et al*, 1996; Smith & Kelly, 1997; Starkweather & Gottwald, 1990; Wall & Myers, 1995).

Our multifactorial model (Figure 1.1) attempts to integrate current research and clinical expertise. Our view is that predisposing physiological and linguistic (speech and language) factors are likely to be significant in the onset and development of stammering, and it is the interaction of these with psychological and environmental aspects that contributes to the severity and persistence of the disorder, as well as the impact it has on a child and the family. For each child there will be an individual combination of factors that contribute to his vulnerability to stammering and the likely prognosis.

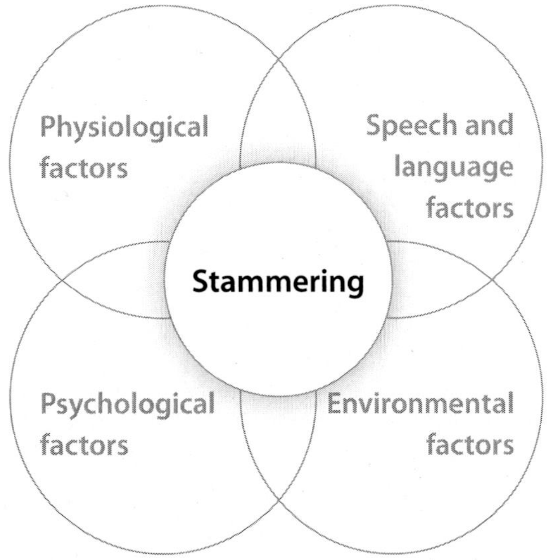

FIGURE 1.1 The multifactorial model

This section will present and discuss the research and the clinical expertise which has influenced the development of the multifactorial model.

Physiological and linguistic (speech and language) factors

Research has explored the following.

Genetics

Stammering has a genetic basis

There is now strong evidence that stammering is more prevalent in families where there is an existing family history (Howie, 1981; Kidd *et al*, 1978; Kloth *et al*, 1999), suggesting a genetic basis to the disorder. In other words, a child inherits 'something' that makes it more likely that he will start to stammer. Studies are currently under way which aim to identify the specific gene or genes or linkages that predispose children to the disorder and, ultimately, to learn why and how they affect a child's fluency (Cox *et al*, 2000; Drayna, 1997; Yairi & Ambrose, 2005). Despite emerging evidence of a genetic component, a family history alone will not determine whether a child might stammer (Farber, 1981; Starkweather, 2002). Starkweather (2002, p.275) argues that genes only increase the likelihood that a behaviour will occur; it is the environment or context which influences the 'extent to which a behavioural trait finds expression'.

The pattern of history in a family also seems to be important. Yairi and Ambrose (2005) found an increased likelihood of 'natural recovery' when a child had a family history of relatives having recovered, whereas a child with a family history of persistent stammering was at increased risk of it persisting.

Clinical implications

Knowledge of the pattern of the family history of stammering will inform our clinical decision-making. It is helpful for parents to understand the possible role of genetic factors in the onset and development of their child's stammer. This is of particular importance for parents who have a tendency to blame themselves or have feelings of guilt about their role in their child's stammering. It is important to address such feelings as these can interfere with the therapy process and prevent parents from making changes (Biggart et al*, 2007; Douglas, 2005).*

Neurological factors

Structural and/or functional differences in the brains of adults who stammer

Studies suggest that stammering is related to underlying structural or functional differences, or both, in the brains of people who stammer compared with fluent controls subjects, which may be governed genetically (Foundas *et al*, 2001; Sommer *et al*, 2002; Watkins *et al*, 2007). Structural differences have been identified in the left rolandic operculum, the area related to the sensorimotor integration that is necessary for fluent speech (Sommer *et al*, 2002) and within the planum temporale, affecting the communication between areas important for auditory perception and motor control of speech (Foundas *et al*, 2001). Although there is considerable variability among the findings of imaging studies, there is general consensus that individuals who stammer exhibit an over activation in right-hemisphere structures that corresponds to left hemispheric activations in speech and language areas in fluent speakers (Braun *et al*, 1997; De Nil *et al*, 2000; Fox *et al*, 1996). In addition, a number of studies have found a lack of activity in the left auditory cortex of individuals who stammer compared with fluent controls subjects (Braun *et al*, 1997; Fox *et al*, 2000; De Nil *et al*, 2003; Neumann *et al*, 2000).

However, these differences have only been identified in teenagers (from the age of 14 years) and adults who stammer, and have not yet been replicated in young children who stammer. It is therefore not yet possible to determine whether these differences are responsible for the onset of stammering or have developed in response to it. It has been suggested that these underlying differences in neurological functioning may be disrupting the complex two-way interaction between language planning and motor processing in people who stammer (see Caruso *et al*, 1999; Ingham & Riley, 1998; Peters *et al*, 2000).

Interestingly, an increased incidence of stammering has been found among children with some degree of brain damage (Poulos & Webster, 1991), with Down's Syndrome (Bloodstein, 1995) or who have been premature (Jennische & Sedin, 1999).

> **Clinical implications**
> *Whilst we do not go into this in detail, it is helpful for parents to understand that predisposing neurological factors may have contributed to the onset and development of their child's stammering.*

Speech motor skills

Differences in speech motor skills

As described above, although brain structure and functioning studies have not yet been conducted with young children, their speech motor skills have been investigated. These studies have found that CWS may have reduced oro-motor skills (Kelly *et al*, 1995; Riley & Riley, 1980), slower response times during both vocal and manual tasks (Bishop *et al*, 1991) and difficulty stabilising and controlling laryngeal movements even during perceptually fluent speech (Conture *et al*, 1986).

> **Clinical implications**
> *These differences in the speech motor skills of CWS may be 'sub-clinical' and may not necessarily be evident when assessing them with the typical clinical measures. It is helpful for parents to understand that a child's speech motor skills may be affecting their ability to be fluent.*

Gender

Boys are more likely than girls to have a speech and/or language problem

Research indicates that there are more boys who persist in stammering than girls (Kloth *et al*, 1999; Yairi & Ambrose 1999). The ratio of boys to girls is reported to be 1:1 close to onset (Yairi, 1983) and by the age of 10 years is 5:1 or 6:1 (Bloodstein & Bernstein Ratner, 2007).

Clinical implications

Gender alone will not influence our clinical decision-making, but is considered along with other information collected about the child to gain an understanding of why they may have started to stammer and their risk of persistence. Interestingly, boys generally show more developmental problems compared with girls and, in particular, are more likely to have difficulties with their speech and language development.

Language skills

Stammering generally emerges at a time of rapid speech and language development, and numerous research studies have attempted to establish a relationship between the two. Some children start to stammer as soon as they start to link words together, whereas others appear to have normal fluency for some time before this breaks down (Kloth *et al*, 1995a).

Research has so far been unable to identify consistent differences in the overall language abilities of CWS compared with fluent control subjects (see Bernstein Ratner 1997a; Nippold, 1990). Some studies have suggested that CWS have less well developed language abilities compared with children who do not stammer (CWNS) (Anderson & Conture, 2000; Byrd & Cooper, 1989; Ratner & Silverman, 2000; Ryan, 1992; Silverman & Ratner, 2002), although the CWS still perform within the normal range. This has led to suggestions that CWS do not present with clinically significant delayed or disordered language but subtle, 'sub-clinical' differences in language ability (see Ratner & Silverman, 2000; Silverman & Ratner, 2002). Similar observations were made earlier regarding a child's speech motor skills. Other studies have either reported no differences between the language skills of CWS and CWNS (Howell *et al*, 2003; Kloth *et al*, 1995a, 1998, 1999) or suggest that CWS may have above-average abilities compared with CWNS (Rommel *et al*, 1999; Watkins *et al*, 1999).

Children who stammer may:

- *have delayed or advanced language skills*
- *present with mismatches in their speech and language skills*

In addition, there are also some data emerging to suggest that CWS are more likely to exhibit discrepancies or mismatches across and between linguistic domains compared to CWNS (Anderson & Conture, 2000; Anderson *et al*, 2005; Bernstein Ratner, 1997b). Anderson *et al* (2005) refer to these discrepancies or mismatches as 'dissociations'. They assessed the expressive and receptive language and phonological skills of CWS and fluent control subjects, and found that CWS are three times more likely to exhibit dissociations across speech and language domains than their fluent peers. The authors (2005, p.242) conclude that 'it is the child's attempt to reconcile or manage these dissociations in speech and language that contributes to disruptions in their speech and language production, which in combination with a genetic predisposition towards stuttering or, perhaps a temperamental disposition that is relatively intolerant of any such disruptions, results in the emergence of persistent stuttering'. They suggest that more attention, effort or resources may be needed to manage these dissociations, and therefore fewer resources are available to establish or maintain fluent speech.

> **Clinical implications**
> *CWS show high variability in their language abilities. The child's language skills may be age-appropriate, delayed or above age level, or he may present with mismatches in his speech and language skills. We need to routinely assess the language skills of each child who stammers. Language difficulties may be subtle and not indicative of clinically significant language delay or disorder.*

Phonological skills

A relationship between phonology and stammering

Although some studies have reported a high proportion of CWS as having speech sound impairments compared with CWNS (Blood *et al*, 2003; Louko *et al*, 1990; Pellowski *et al*, 2000), Nippold (1990, 2002) has identified a number of methodological weaknesses in these studies and suggests that further study is needed to ascertain how frequently stammering and phonological disorders co-occur. Paden *et al* (1999) demonstrated an association between phonological skills and persistence of stammering. In their study, children showed great individual variability in their phonological ability, but as a group children with poorer phonological skills at the onset of stammering were more likely to persist than those with age-appropriate skills.

> **Clinical implications**
> *We need to routinely assess a child's phonological skills and collect information about the history of a child's phonological development, in particular their skills at the time of the onset of stammering.*

Linguistic context and stammering

Increased stammering on longer and more complex sentences

Moments of stammering have been found to be influenced by a number of linguistic variables. Stammering tends to occur at the beginning of an utterance (Silverman, 1974), at clause boundaries (Howell & Au-Yeung, 1995; Wall *et al*, 1981) and on function words rather than content words (Howell *et al*, 1999). Stammering also tends to be more frequent on longer and more syntactically complex sentences (Bernstein Ratner & Sih, 1987; Gaines *et al*,

1991; Kadi-Hanifi & Howell, 1992; Logan & Conture, 1995; Melnick & Conture, 2000). It is important to note that these associations are not true for all CWS (Yaruss, 1999).

> ***Clinical implications***
> *If the use of longer and more syntactically complex sentences is affecting a child's ability to be fluent, we take this into account when considering what the child may need to help him be more fluent.*

Bilingualism

Stammering is not more prevalent in bilingual speakers

Systematic research on the relationship between stammering and bilingualism is limited (see Van Borsel *et al*, 2001). Although earlier studies suggested that stammering is more prevalent in bilingual speakers (Stern, 1948; Travis *et al*, 1937), a more recent study reported that stammering is as likely in bilingual speakers as in monolingual speakers (Au-Yeung *et al*, 2000). We need further research to explore any potential association between stammering and bilingualism.

> ***Clinical implications***
> *Limited advice is available to SLTs about the assessment and treatment of stammering in bilingual children. Although, in the past, SLTs advised parents to limit the number of languages spoken to their child who stammers, or to avoid code switching, this advice is no longer considered appropriate. We need to ascertain as far as possible the child's level of proficiency in the languages he speaks to identify whether there is a difficulty in learning both the home language and English, or a difficulty in learning English as a second language.*

In the next section, we will consider environmental and psychological factors. In our view these do not contribute to the onset of stammering, but interact with predisposing physiological and linguistic (speech and language) factors, contributing to how a child's stammer develops in terms of its severity and persistence as well as the impact it has on a child and the family.

Environmental and psychological factors

Communicative environment

The research is very clear that there is no evidence that the communication and interaction styles of parents of CWS and CWNS are different (for a review see Nippold & Rudzinski, 1995) or that they have a role in the onset of stammering (Kloth *et al*, 1995b). However, some researchers are beginning to speculate that the underlying vulnerabilities that predispose children to stammer also make it more difficult for them to be fluent in the context of typical adult–child interactions (Felsenfeld, 1997; Miles & Bernstein Ratner, 2001). There is also a suggestion that stammering may result in a change in the interaction style of parents (Kloth *et al*, 1998; Meyers & Freeman, 1985a, 1985b), perhaps as a consequence of the increased anxiety induced by the stammering (Zenner *et al*, 1978). Importantly, while there is no association with stammering onset, there is some evidence that changes to parent interaction styles can have an influence on the frequency of stammering for some children, although any long-term impact has yet to be adequately demonstrated (Guitar *et al*, 1992; Guitar & Marchinkoski, 2001; Newman & Smit, 1989; Winslow & Guitar, 1994).

Clinical implications

The research findings on the role of parents' communication and interaction styles have influenced the development of Palin PCI and contribute to our rationale for involving parents in therapy for young CWS.

Parents' anxiety

Stammering
↑ ↓
Parental anxiety

Although there is no research evidence about the effect of parental anxiety on stammering, parents have been found to be more anxious when interacting with a CWS than a CWNS (Zenner *et al*, 1978). If a parent is very worried, the child may pick up on this and respond to it (Douglas, 2005). We would speculate that the reaction a child gets when he stammers may affect his awareness and attitude to his speech.

Anxiety can affect how parents react to their child (Biggart *et al*, 2007; Douglas, 2005), with parenting tending to be less consistent when parents are feeling very emotional (Allen & Rapee, 2005). Sleeping and eating difficulties in young children in particular may have a negative effect on parents' self-esteem and confidence in managing their child (Douglas, 2005), and difficulties in managing a child's problems generally can cause some parents to question their parenting skills (Schmidt, 2005).

Clinical implications

Families are regarded as systems of interconnected and interdependent individuals, with each family member's behaviour affecting the others in a circular manner. Family members affect one another's thoughts, feelings and actions, and a change in one person's functioning is inevitably followed by reciprocal changes in the functioning of others (Epstein & Bishop, 1981). Therefore, the child who stammers needs to be considered within the context of the family system.

It is important not to ignore parents' natural anxiety, and it is our experience that when parents have a good understanding of stammering and the role they have in supporting their child, their anxiety is reduced. Some parents are aware that they respond differently to sleeping, eating and behavioural issues because of their worry about exacerbating the stammer. We therefore help parents, where appropriate, to recognise and understand how their own emotional state may affect their responses to the child's behaviour, and we provide alternative strategies for managing any difficulties they report. This allows parents to make changes that enable them to manage the child in a more consistent way and to respond to the child rather than the stammering.

Temperament

Recent years have seen a renewed focus placed on the relationship between stammering and temperament (see Conture, 2001; Guitar, 1998). Although there is no suggestion that particular temperament characteristics account for the onset of stammering, it has been proposed that temperament may play a role in how the problem develops.

Studies have shown that compared to fluent children, young CWS are:

Temperament may play a role in the development of stammering

- more active and less able to maintain and shift attention (Embrechts *et al*, 2000; Karrass *et al*, 2006; Nicholas *et al*, 2006)
- less distractible and more vigilant (Anderson *et al*, 2003)
- more impulsive (Embrechts *et al*, 2000)
- less adaptable to change, differences and new situations (Embrechts *et al*, 2000; Anderson *et al*, 2003)
- more reactive to environmental stimuli: they become more intensely aroused when faced with everyday stressful, challenging or exciting situations (Karrass *et al*, 2006; Wakaba, 1998)
- less able to regulate their emotions: once they become upset or excited they are less able to return to a calmer state (Karrass *et al*, 2006)
- more anxious, introverted, sensitive, withdrawn, shy, insecure, fearful and less likely to take risks (Fowlie & Cooper, 1978; Nicholas *et al*, 2006; Oyler, 1996; Oyler & Ramig, 1995).

Karrass *et al* (2006) have hypothesised that these characteristics may play a role in the development of stammering. For example, CWS with a more reactive temperament may be more aware, and therefore become more concerned about, the episodes of stammering in their speech. In turn, if they generally find it hard to regulate their emotions, these concerns may result in further stammering. In addition, CWS identified as having difficulties with attention control may find it harder to shift their attention and 'to move on' or 'let go' when they have been less fluent.

> ***Clinical implications***
> *Within the clinic, parents frequently describe their child who stammers as being 'highly sensitive', 'easily upset' and 'a bit of a worrier'. In addition, they are often observed to be children who 'set themselves high standards', are 'perfectionists' and 'like to get things right'. We consider how each child's individual temperament may be having an effect on his stammer and how he is managing it*

Child's awareness

A young CWS may be aware of his stammer

From the age of three years both CWS and normally fluent children can recognise that stammered speech is different from fluent speech (Ambrose & Yairi, 1994; Ezrati-Vinacour *et al*, 2001). Not only do CWS as young as three or four years of age have an awareness of stammered speech, but they also are more likely than gender-matched fluent control subjects to have a negative attitude towards their speech (Vanryckeghem *et al*, 2005). In addition, it has also been shown that the attitude of CWS towards their speech becomes increasingly negative as they get older (Vanryckeghem & Brutten, 1997).

> ***Clinical implications***
> *Although not all young CWS will show awareness of their stammering, we routinely evaluate the awareness and attitudes of young CWS during assessment, and therapy may need to address any identified negative attitudes.*

Summary

The multifactorial model combines research evidence with clinical expertise to identify issues which are relevant in the onset, development and persistence of stammering. The multifactorial model provides a framework which informs our assessment procedure and our therapy decisions for each individual child and his family. It can also be used to explain to parents the unique combination of factors that may contribute to the onset and subsequent development of their child's stammering.

Wider application of the multifactorial model

This model may be used to understand a variety of different disorders that present in an SLT clinic. Identifying the various physiological, linguistic (speech and language), environmental and psychological factors which may be significant for a child with, for example, specific language impairment (SLI), a voice disorder or phonological difficulties, may help the SLT and the child's parents to gain a better understanding of the problem and its remediation.

Which children are more likely to grow out of early stammering?

In the past, the focus of an assessment of a young dysfluent child was to distinguish between early stammering and 'normal non-fluency'. Although many practitioners provide clinical guidelines on differential diagnosis, this is generally viewed as a challenge owing to the overlap between the two groups (Ambrose & Yairi, 1999; Conture, 1990; Curlee, 1999).

We would argue that if a child is referred because of concern about his fluency, this child should be viewed as stammering. The amount and type of stammering heard in a child's speech has clearly triggered the attention of a parent or an early years practitioner, and a referral has subsequently been made. In fact, in a file audit of more than 1,000 children brought to a specialist stammering clinic, only 0.9 per cent of parents were found to incorrectly identify their child's speech as being a stammering problem (Onslow, 2004).

Approximately 75 per cent of children who experience stammering will resolve the problem naturally (Johannsen, 2000; Kloth *et al*, 1999; Mansson, 2000; Yairi & Ambrose, 1999). The challenge for SLTs therefore is to identify those children who are likely to recover naturally and those who are at risk of persistence, and to ensure that resources are allocated appropriately to those who need them.

In the last 10 to 15 years the findings of three major longitudinal studies have contributed to our knowledge about which factors may be associated with recovery and persistence in young CWS (Johannsen, 2000; Kloth *et al*, 1999; Yairi & Ambrose, 1999). In these studies, the progress of a large number of children has been monitored over a number of years, and comparisons have been made across a range of variables between those children who recovered and those who continued to stammer.

These studies have observed the progress of different subpopulations of CWS, as follows.

- Children who have a parent who stammers (Kloth *et al*, 1999). The children were monitored before stammering had actually begun and so findings have informed us about the variables which influence onset, as well as those that influence recovery.
- Children who were referred to an SLT clinic (Johannsen, 2000). The children in this study most closely reflect the clinical population, as they were referred because of concern about their stammering, rather than for inclusion in a study. The majority had therapy during the course of the study and the findings therefore reflect factors which influence prognosis both with and without therapy.
- Children who were referred to a research study close to the onset of stammering (Yairi & Ambrose, 1999). In this study, children were recruited from preschool settings and through advertisements. These children were not necessarily referred as a result of parents' or professionals' concerns about their speech. This was therefore not a clinical population of CWS. Although there was no therapy available as part of the study, parents were able to obtain therapy through other channels. It should therefore be assumed that the results reflect a population containing some children who have received therapy as well as some who have not.

It is important to understand the differences between the subpopulations of the studies in order to interpret and apply the research findings appropriately to our own clinical populations.

We will now summarise the key findings from the three different research studies highlighting the factors which have influenced our clinical decisions about recovery and persistence.

Family history of stammering

According to Yairi and Ambrose (2005) a child's family history of stammering is the single most reliable predictor of persistence for children just beginning to stammer. These authors state that a positive family history alone is not sufficient for predicting outcome, rather it is the *pattern* of history that is key. A child with a family history of persistent stammering is at increased risk of continuing to stammer, whereas a child with a family history of relatives having recovered has a greater chance of recovering.

Is there a family history of stammering?
Did they recover or persist?

The role of family history in recovery and persistence varied for Rommel *et al* (1999) depending on when recovery took place. These authors did not find a relationship between a positive family history and persistence for those children whom they described as recovering early (within 18 months of being recruited into their study). However, when they compared those who recovered later (between 18 and 54 months after being recruited into the study) with those whose stammering persisted, children with more members of the family having a history of stammering were more likely to persist. They did not specify whether the family history was of recovery or persistence.

Clinical implications

When we are considering risk factors for persistence we need to collect information about family history of stammering, both in the immediate and extended family, and to ask whether the history was of recovery or persistence.

Gender

More girls recover than boys

A higher proportion of girls recover than boys, although the difference has not been found to be statistically significant (Johannsen, 2000; Kloth *et al*, 1999; Yairi & Ambrose, 1999). Interestingly, girls have been found to recover at an earlier age than boys (Yairi *et al*, 1996).

Clinical implications

Overall, the trend is towards a girl being more likely to recover than a boy.

Age at onset

Although the difference was not significant, Yairi *et al* (1996) found that children in the persistent stammering group tended to be older at onset (age three years and over), whereas Johannsen (2000) found that children who were younger at onset (under age three years) were more likely to persist.

Clinical implications

Given the conflicting findings, age of onset may not be a clear indicator of vulnerability.

Length of time since onset of stammering

If the child has been stammering for more than 12 months, he is more likely to persist

The majority of children have been found to recover within the first 12 to 18 months after stammering begins (Yairi & Ambrose, 1992a; Yairi *et al*, 1996). Although some children will still achieve fluency after this (Yairi & Ambrose, 1999), the probability of recovery has been found to decrease with the length of time they have been stammering (Yairi *et al*, 1996).

Clinical implications

We collect information about length of time since onset of the child's stammering. Even if it is a fluctuating pattern, a child who has already been stammering for 12 months is at increased risk of persistence.

Pattern of change in stammering over time

If the child's stammer is improving, he is more likely to recover

Children whose stammering has reduced over time have been shown to be more likely to recover, while children demonstrating a stable level of stammering or an increase in stammering over time have been found to be at a higher risk of having a persistent problem (Johannsen, 2000; Yairi & Ambrose, 1999; Yairi *et al*, 1996). The children who were most likely to persist were those whose secondary behaviours (such as head movements) stayed the same or increased in number or severity within the first year of onset. (Yairi & Ambrose, 2005; Yairi *et al*, 1993). An increase in the proportion of prolongations in a child's speech was also found to be an indicator of higher risk, along with the continuing presence of multiple repetitions (ie containing three or more repetitions, for example, *ba-ba-ba-bag*), over time (Yairi & Ambrose, 2005). Children who recovered tended to show a reduction in secondary behaviours, the proportion of prolongations in their speech reduced and they did not continue to show multiple repetitions over time.

Clinical implications

At assessment we collect information about how the stammering has changed over time, both in terms of its frequency and the type of stammering behaviours observed. We may need to demonstrate to parents the different types of stammering behaviours found in a child's speech, including avoidance, to help them make this judgement. If parents report a fluctuating pattern over time, we ask them to describe the overall trend. If the stammering is improving the child is more likely to recover.

Phonological skills

Phonological delay at time of onset may be a risk factor

Great individual variability has been found in the phonological abilities of both children who recovered and those who continued to stammer. However, when assessed close to stammering onset, children in the persistent group have been found to have delayed phonological skills (rather than disordered) compared with the children in the recovered group, a difference that was no longer evident one year post-onset (Paden & Yairi, 1996; Paden *et al*, 1999; Yairi *et al*, 1996).

Clinical implications

We collect information about the history of a child's phonological development, in particular his phonological skills at the time of the onset of stammering, as well as carry out an informal or formal assessment of his phonological skills at assessment. Evidence of phonological delay during the first year of stammering suggests increased risk of persistence.

Language skills

The role of children's language skills in persistence and recovery is not clear. Kloth *et al* (1995b) did not find any differences in the receptive or expressive language skills of children who began to stammer, compared with those who remained fluent. In addition, no differences were found when the receptive and expressive language skills of the children who persisted were compared with those who recovered (Kloth *et al*, 1999).

Delayed or advanced language may be a risk factor for persistence

In contrast, Rommel (2000) and Hage (2000) found that children in the persistent group had higher vocabulary scores compared with the children in the recovered group and they tended to use longer words and produce longer sentences at an increased speed. In other words they demonstrated advanced language skills relative to matched peers.

The findings of Yairi and colleagues have varied over time. Their early investigations of language skills indicated that children who persisted had lower language scores than those who recovered (Yairi *et al*, 1996), yet later studies (Watkins & Yairi, 1997; Watkins *et al*, 1999), suggest that there are no differences in the language skills of those who recover and those who persist. More recent studies by Watkins (2005) and Watkins and Johnson (2004) have focused on children who presented with advanced expressive language skills close to the onset of stammering. When these children were followed up four years post-onset, it was found that the children who were still stammering had maintained advanced expressive language skills over time, whereas the language skills of those who recovered moved from an advanced pattern to one that was more age-appropriate over time. This suggests that language change may be associated with recovery in children who have advanced skills. This pattern of change has also been found in the language skills of children following the Lidcombe Program (Bonelli *et al*, 2000).

> ***Clinical implications***
> *We need to, informally and formally, assess a child's language as part of our assessment. Although the findings have been conflicting, we view delayed or advanced language skills as complicating the stammer, and therefore predictive of vulnerability to persistence.*

Severity of stammering

Severity of stammering does not necessarily indicate prognosis

Yairi and colleagues did not find that severity of stammering (as measured by the frequency of stammering) was predictive of outcome (Yairi *et al*, 1996; Yairi & Ambrose, 1999). Indeed, they found that, during the first few months of stammering, children who later recovered were stammering as severely as, or even more severely than, those who persisted. Children who initially present with mild stammering are therefore not necessarily those who will recover, and severe stammering does not rule out recovery.

In contrast, although Johannsen (2000) found considerable individual variation in severity in both the recovered and persistent groups, she found that the prognosis was better for children with less severe stammering.

> ***Clinical implications***
> *We assess the severity of stammering in a child's speech during assessment; however, other factors need to be considered when deciding whether or not to intervene. Mild stammering is not necessarily evidence of recovery and severe stammering does not indicate persistence.*

Conclusions

Although the findings of the above research studies have been influential in shaping our clinical decision-making in recent years, it is not possible to predict with 100 per cent certainty the prognosis for any individual child. No single factor is necessarily sufficient to predict outcome and to date there has been no attempt to investigate the impact of coexisting factors, or to determine whether one factor has greater influence over persistence than another.

Furthermore, these research findings must be considered in the light of clinical experience. We recommend that if a child or his parents, or both, are highly anxious about his speech and it is causing them distress, a full assessment is arranged, even if no risk factors for persistence are identified.

What is Palin PCI?

Many treatment approaches for early stammering involve either an *indirect* or a *direct* component, or a combination of both *indirect* and *direct* methods (Conture, 2001; Guitar, 2006; Gottwald & Starkweather, 1995; Onslow *et al*, 2003; Starkweather & Gottwald, 1990; Stewart & Turnbull, 2007; Wall & Myers, 1995; Yaruss *et al*, 2006). The *indirect* component typically involves making changes in the child's environment and, in particular, modifications to parents' interaction styles in the belief that this will facilitate a child's fluency. The *direct* therapy component usually involves a child being asked to make specific changes to his speech production, such as slowing his speech rate or using a gradual onset to words (Meyers & Woodford, 1992; Runyan & Runyan, 1999). Alternatively, operant methods are used to acknowledge and reinforce fluent speech, and to acknowledge and correct stammered speech (Onslow *et al*, 2003).

Palin PCI:

- *Interaction strategies*
- *Family strategies*
- *Child strategies*

Palin PCI therapy is a combined *indirect* and *direct* treatment approach for the young child who stammers (aged seven years and under). Parents are a key component of the approach. We begin with a comprehensive assessment which enables us to develop an individualised treatment programme using the specific information gained about the child's abilities and underlying vulnerabilities within the context of the family. This individualised programme of therapy will typically consist of two or more of the following three main strands.

- *Interaction strategies*: these may include following the child's lead, using a balance of comments and questions, and use of pausing.
- *Family strategies*: these may include confidence-building, behaviour management, turn-taking, and dealing with feelings.
- *Child strategies*: these may include *direct* speech modification strategies, such as slowing down and making use of pausing.

The programme is initially delivered as a six-week package of therapy, followed by a six-week home consolidation period. After this time, the child's progress is reviewed and further decisions are made about the need for ongoing therapy and what form this should take.

The programme is flexible and adapted according to each child's individual and changing needs. For some children, the outcome is fluency within normal limits, whereas for others strategies are established to support their fluency and to minimise the impact of the stammering on both the child and the family.

We will now describe how Palin PCI evolved to its current form and the various influences, including research, which have shaped it over the years.

Early PCI

We first implemented PCI in the 1980s (Rustin, 1987) and it was published in its most detailed form in 1996 (Rustin *et al*, 1996). The programme evolved during the 'wait and see' period, when limited information was available to make a differential diagnosis between those children who were likely to recover without therapy and those who were not. This meant that there was a tendency to provide parents with advice 'to tide them over' until the picture became clearer. Even when the child presented with a severe stammer and was expressing concern, there was a legacy (now discredited) of nervousness within the profession about drawing the child's attention to his stammer or acknowledging the difficulty the child was experiencing.

Early PCI: teaching parents what not to do

Treatment therefore tended to comprise advice to parents, typically a list of 'dos and don'ts', for example telling the parents to slow down their own speech, not to interrupt the child, not to ask too many questions and not to finish the child's sentence for him. We realised how difficult it is to change one's habitual behaviour from a list of 'dos and don'ts' and we developed PCI as a way of helping parents to put this advice into practice.

Across the profession at this time, children were usually seen individually while parents stayed outside in a waiting room. Thus the involvement of parents was unusual and innovative, largely due to the vision and drive of the late Dr Lena Rustin, who headed the team. We recognised the central role of parents in helping their children and we wanted to alleviate their anxiety about the stammering by giving concrete help rather than vague reassurances and sometimes conflicting advice.

In those early days, SLTs were generally working within the framework of the 'medical model' and behaviour therapy was strongly influential. The emphasis of the early form of PCI was on the expert clinician *teaching* and *training* parents what *not* to do in order to reduce their child's stammering. The clinician and the parents together would analyse the interaction styles to identify patterns which might be 'undermining' the child's ability to speak fluently. This focus on what parents were doing that was unhelpful reflected the trend of research studies at this time, which compared the interaction styles of the parents of CWS and the parents of CWNS. Research findings were often expressed in negative terms, with the parents of CWS described as being more negative interactors (Kasprisin Burrelli *et al*, 1972), making more demands, commands and requests of their children (Langlois *et al*, 1986), and interrupting more and failing to allow the child to answer questions (Mordecai, 1979) compared with the parents of fluent children. Advice sheets and clinical texts popular at this time are in line with these research findings (Irwin, 1988; Rustin *et al*, 1996). The subplot of these texts seemed to suggest that parents were at fault, even while we were telling them that there was no evidence that parents caused their children to stammer. Thus, although PCI in its early form was addressing some of the shortfalls in the management of early stammering, it may also have inadvertently increased parents' feelings of guilt.

Early PCI was commonly misperceived as a purely *indirect* approach to the management of stammering, which followed the Johnsonian (Johnson, 1942) directive that parents should not draw the child's attention to his stammering. In fact, from the outset, PCI promoted the position that stammering should be openly acknowledged and discussed, and that there should not be a 'conspiracy of silence' (Rustin & Cook, 1995). In their early description of the PCI approach, Botterill *et al* (1991) strongly advocated that parents acknowledge the child's difficulty and maintain an open dialogue with the child about it. Furthermore, PCI also included a component of *direct* speech modification with the child, focusing on developing his cognitive awareness of how to facilitate his own natural fluency, largely based on *The Fluency Development System for Young Children* (Meyers & Woodford, 1992). PCI therefore combined *indirect* and *direct* methods to manage the child's stammering in a comprehensive programme.

Over time, we have reflected on our PCI programme and adapted it, in light of new research and the changing trend in clinical practice, from the previous behavioural methods to the counselling approach, which starts with the client's viewpoint. This has led to significant changes between the original programme and the current Palin PCI, both in terms of its rationale and the way the programme is implemented.

The current Palin PCI programme

The principles and supporting research are as follows.

Parents of CWS are viewed as interacting with their child in many ways that support his fluency

Parents are already supporting their child's fluency

Parents often already know what seems to affect their child's fluency and respond instinctively to this, for example by helping him to calm down, take his time and so on. The therapy process elicits and builds on this knowledge, addressing parents' fears about whether they are doing the right things. There has therefore been a major shift in focus from what the parents need to 'stop doing', to what the parents are already doing naturally to help their child. Therapy reinforces parents' ability to interact in ways that match the child's fluency needs, and focuses on increasing these helpful interactions in the home environment. This shift in focus reduces the likelihood of parents blaming themselves.

Parents of CWS are not regarded as being different from parents of CWNS in terms of their interaction style

Parents of CWS have normal interaction styles

This principle is supported by research findings (for a review see Nippold & Rudzinski, 1995). The parents of CWS are no different from the parents of CWNS in terms of their rate of speech (Kelly, 1994a, 1994b; Meyers & Freeman, 1985a; Yaruss & Conture, 1995; Zebrowski, 1995), response time latencies (Zebrowski, 1995), interrupting behaviours (Kelly, 1994a, 1994b; Kelly & Conture, 1992; Meyers & Freeman, 1985b), levels of assertiveness and responsiveness (Weiss & Zebrowski, 1991) or their interaction styles (Embrechts & Ebben, 1999).

Parental interaction styles can be modified and these changes can improve fluency

Interactions may be changed and can increase fluency

Palin PCI is based on the premise that interaction is a two-way process and each person influences the other. Some studies have found that children's stammering significantly reduces when parents slow down their rate of speech (Guitar *et al*, 1992; Guitar & Marchinkoski, 2001), increase their response time latency (Newman & Smit, 1989) and establish structured turn-taking (Winslow & Guitar, 1994). Importantly, though, the impact of these changes made by parents is not consistent for all CWS (Zebrowski *et al*, 1996), highlighting the importance of therapy being individually tailored, based on each child's particular needs. During the course of the Palin PCI programme we therefore monitor whether an interaction style is having the necessary effect and make adjustments as required.

Stammering influences parents' interaction styles

Stammering can affect parents' interaction

Not only is there some evidence that modifications in a parent's interaction style can reduce the frequency of stammering but there is also evidence that stammering influences parents' interaction styles (Meyers & Freeman, 1985a, 1985b; Zenner *et al*, 1978). The mothers of both CWS and CWNS have been found to use a faster rate of speech (Meyers & Freeman, 1985b), interrupt more frequently (Meyers & Freeman, 1985a) and are more anxious (Zenner *et al*, 1978) when interacting with CWS compared with CWNS. It is possible that these altered interaction styles are a result of increased anxiety associated with the stammering.

In their longitudinal study of children at risk of stammering due to a family history, Kloth and colleagues (1995a, 1995b, 1998, 1999) found that parents may change their interaction style in response to a child's stammering. These authors found that, before stammering begins, there were no differences in the behaviours of mothers whose children started to stammer and those whose children did not (Kloth *et al*, 1995b). However, four years later, it was found that mothers of the children who persisted in stammering had changed their interaction style, exerting more *direct* pressure on the children to respond verbally than they did before onset (Kloth *et al*, 1999). The mothers were described as using a style which was more intervening than before, with more turn-exchanges, more requests for information and more affirmatives. The mothers of children whose stammering resolved did not change their style. Clearly, these findings do not support the notion that parents' behaviours result in the onset of stammering. On the contrary, they suggest that parents changed their interaction styles in response to the child's stammering. It is important to note, however, that the children included in this study all had at least one parent who stammered, which may have influenced their response to the stammering.

The underlying vulnerabilities that predispose a child to stammer may also make it more difficult for him to be fluent in the context of typical adult–child interactions

The child's vulnerabilities may make it harder for him to cope in a normal interaction

Although the input of parents of CWS has been found to be the same as that of parents of CWNS, it is possible that if a child has underlying linguistic vulnerabilities it may make it harder for him to assimilate or respond to parental input (Miles & Bernstein Ratner, 2001). Another suggestion is that a child's temperament may influence how he responds to different parental interaction styles. Felsenfeld (1997) suggests that a child who has a highly reactive temperament may be more responsive to a parent's fast rate of speech, particularly at the age when stammering typically begins. Individual children may therefore respond differently to particular interaction styles.

Similarities and differences between the Palin PCI programme and other treatment approaches for early stammering

Indirect therapy as the first stage of management

As previously mentioned, Palin PCI consists of both *indirect* (interaction and family strategies) and *direct* components (child strategies). As with many other approaches (Conture, 2001; Conture & Melnick, 1999; Yaruss *et al*, 2006), we recommend the *indirect* component of Palin PCI as the first stage of management, followed by more *direct* methods. We consider that the *indirect* therapy component will be sufficient to help most children to achieve fluency (Millard *et al*, 2008). For those who continue to stammer, parents have established strategies which support the child's fluency and minimise the impact of the stammering, while laying the foundations for future *direct* therapy with the child. We have found that the insight, knowledge and skills gained by parents during the assessment and the *indirect* component of the programme play an important role in helping the child to transfer the speech management skills they learn during the *direct* therapy stage of the programme. The *direct* therapy component of Palin PCI has been developed over a number of years, and is based on the Meyers and Woodford (1992) programme. Since being trained in the approach, we also sometimes use the Lidcombe Program (Onslow *et al*, 2003) as a *direct* method.

Parents select their own targets

There are many similarities between the Palin PCI programme and other *indirect* approaches (Conture, 2001; Guitar, 2006; Gottwald & Starkweather, 1995; Starkweather & Gottwald, 1990; Stewart & Turnbull, 2007; Wall & Myers 1995; Yaruss *et al*, 2006) in terms of the interaction strategies selected and the end goal of each strategy. Palin PCI differs from other *indirect* approaches in that there are no standard interaction strategies that all parents work on and in the way that interaction strategies are chosen and implemented.

Parents select their own interaction targets, based on the child's needs

In the majority of other programmes the clinician instructs the parent about the interaction strategy they should adopt and then models the behaviours, which the parent copies and practises (Conture & Melnick, 1999; Guitar, 2006; Starkweather & Gottwald, 1990; Yaruss *et al*, 2006). In Palin PCI we encourage parents to select their own interaction strategies, based on their knowledge about what helps their child. We guide parents through a process of identifying those strategies that they are already using which are helpful for the child's fluency, and developing these strategies further, as appropriate. It is the role of the therapist to elicit the parents' skills and knowledge, and to enhance them further. Palin PCI therefore reinforces the expert, intuitive understanding that parents already have about their child.

Family strategies

A further difference between the Palin PCI programme and other approaches is the inclusion of family strategies as well as interaction strategies. During Palin PCI we help parents deal with concerns such as acknowledging the child's stammer, coping with a sensitive child, confidence-building, and behaviour management such as setting boundaries and routines, turn-taking and bedtimes. Although there is, as yet, no evidence that these areas are directly related to stammering, they are often reported by parents as being stressful and as having an impact on the family, and, in turn, the child's fluency.

Palin PCI therefore differs from other *indirect* approaches in its broad scope. We individualise the programme for each child and family by selecting interaction and family strategies which are felt to be key in further supporting the child's fluency. Palin PCI also differs from other *indirect* approaches in the methods used to select and rehearse the interaction strategies for each family.

The Palin PCI style

What makes therapy work – the therapy content or the therapist?

In the field of psychotherapy and counselling there is an interesting debate about what influences the success of therapy. Wampold (2001) suggests that it is the therapist, rather than the therapy, which makes the difference, and that the specific treatments or techniques account for less than one per cent of variance among patients. Spinelli (1994) suggests that the crucial factor in successful therapy is the 'bond' formed between the therapist and client.

We subscribe to the view that effective therapy lies in the nature of the alliance which is formed with the families. Our work has been influenced by a range of different psychological and counselling approaches, including:

- Solution-focused brief therapy (De Shazer, 1988, 1996; O'Hanlon and Weiner-Davis, 1989)
- Cognitive therapy (Beck, 1995)
- Personal construct psychology (Fransella, 1972; Kelly, 1955)
- Family systems theory (Epstein & Bishop, 1981).

We now place greater emphasis on developing the client-clinician relationship and encouraging parents to utilise and develop their own problem-solving and management skills. Our role is that of facilitator and reinforcer, providing

Our role:
- *facilitator*
- *reinforcer*
- *highlighting strengths*
- *collaborative*

feedback which focuses on strengths. We have a collaborative partnership with parents, which is based on a shared perception of the problem, with clear goals and a shared responsibility.

As previously discussed, a fundamental premise of Palin PCI is that parents instinctively know what seems to help their child who stammers, but often they do not know that they know. Our job is to elicit this intuitive understanding and develop it, thus reducing parents' anxiety about the problem and increasing their confidence in their own ability to manage it.

Does Palin PCI work?

EBP:
- *best research evidence*
- *clinical expertise*
- *patient's values and circumstances*

According to Straus *et al* (2005, p.1), evidence-based practice (EBP) involves 'the integration of best research evidence with our clinical expertise and our patient's unique values and circumstances'. The goal for SLTs is to provide a high-quality EBP service to each individual child and family. In our clinical decision-making, we need to use our clinical knowledge, experience and expertise to evaluate the quality of published research and to consider its appropriateness and application to a particular family.

Research from efficacy to effectiveness

The clinical work at the MPC is informed by a wide range of theoretical and clinical models from the field of psychology as well as speech and language pathology, providing a broad evidence base to support our practices. The MPC has a research programme to investigate the evidence base for Palin PCI. This research programme is based on the model proposed by Robey and Schultz (1998). The model advocates systematically investigating therapy through a progression of levels, moving from treatment efficacy research, where therapy is investigated under optimal conditions (eg implemented by SLTs expert in the application of the therapy programme, in a specifically resourced specialist environment), to treatment effectiveness research, where therapy is investigated under clinical conditions (eg in typical settings for SLTs). As the research progresses through the different levels, the factors that influence outcome are isolated and investigated. There are five phases of research described in a logical series, but which are not discrete.

Phase 1:
Single case study (Matthews et al, *1997)*

In Phase 1, clinical reports, small group studies or single case studies, or both, are used to demonstrate whether there is evidence that a treatment is effective. Clinical reports detailing the positive effect of Palin PCI for individual clients have been available for a number of years (Rustin *et al*, 1996). Matthews *et al* (1997) conducted a more structured single-case systematic investigation of Palin PCI. They monitored the progress of a four-year-old boy for six weeks before therapy, six weeks during therapy and six weeks after therapy. The percentage of words stammered was calculated from speech samples obtained while the child played with each parent in the clinic for a period of 20 minutes, once a week. The therapy resulted in a significant reduction in the frequency of the child's stammering.

In Phase 2 research, studies are designed to define how therapy works, which clients are suitable for a particular programme, the amount of therapy and the method of delivery that will have the greatest impact. Within this phase, outcome measures are also identified. Information from Phase 1 clinical reports, along with findings from other research studies, have contributed to our thinking about the mechanisms involved in Palin PCI and how it works, leading to the development of suggestions for testing in Phase 2.

Six children aged 3:0 – 4:11 years with a wide range of language skills took part in a Phase 3 multiple single-subject study to evaluate the efficacy of Palin PCI therapy. Results indicated that parents are able to make changes in their interaction style during Palin PCI, and that these changes are maintained over time. Specifically, in this group, fathers significantly reduced the proportion of utterances that were requests for information and reduced the length of their turn, while mothers in this study significantly reduced the number of their utterances that were instructions. We have yet to demonstrate whether these changes in parents' interaction styles are directly associated with gains in fluency.

The data were also analysed to investigate the relationship between Palin PCI therapy and child language. Results indicated that children's language continued to develop while they were receiving Palin PCI therapy and for three months post-therapy (Nicholas *et al*, 2004); therefore there was no indication that Palin PCI has a negative impact on language development. An additional five children who began therapy with advanced receptive and expressive language skills (as measured on the *Reynell Developmental Language Scales III: The University of Reading Edition* (Edwards *et al*, 1997)) were found to show a different pattern of development. At six months post-therapy these children had maintained their advanced receptive language skills over time. In contrast, their expressive language skills showed a reduction over time relative to age. These children moved from being advanced to having more age-appropriate expressive language skills at six months post-therapy. This pattern of development has been associated with increased fluency in children who have received minimal intervention (Watkins, 2005; Watkins & Johnson, 2004) and following the Lidcombe Program (Bonelli *et al*, 2000). These findings suggest that some children may be achieving increased fluency by slowing the development of language in a fluency–language trade-off, or may be using simpler language in order to achieve greater fluency.

> **Phase 2:**
> - *PCI and changes in children's language (Nicholas* et al, *2004)*
> - *Development of parent rating scales (Millard, 2002)*

Phase 2 also seeks to identify the appropriate outcome measures for use in effectiveness studies. We propose that these should reflect the multidimensional nature of stammering as well as the expectations and needs of the client. Frequency of stammers (percentage of syllables stammered) is the usual measure of success in therapy for young CWS, but this does not reflect the variability of stammering from day to day or situation to situation and is unlikely to be representative of a child's overall fluency. In addition, we would argue that measures of the frequency of stammering should be supported by an evaluation of the impact of the stammering on the child and the parents. This might include an evaluation of parents' worries about their child's stammer, their confidence in managing it and their knowledge of strategies for managing their child's stammer more effectively. However, there are few assessment tools available that evaluate these broader issues adequately. In an attempt to address this, Millard (2002) conducted a Delphi study to find out what parents consider to be the most important outcomes in therapy and to develop an outcome measurement tool for parents who receive Palin PCI therapy. A group of parents who had attended the MPC for Palin PCI therapy with their children during the previous year selected the following as important targets of the therapy programme: stammering frequency and severity; the child's anxiety, frustration and concern about speech; confidence in speaking and turn-taking skills; parents' own level of concern; confidence in managing the stammering effectively; and the impact on the family as a whole. A series of rating scales was subsequently developed for use before, during and after therapy to evaluate change.

Phase 3 of the research framework relates to large-scale efficacy research. Randomised controlled trials (RCTs) are generally viewed as the 'gold standard' methodology for treatment efficacy research (Jones *et al,* 2001). However, there are practical and methodological limitations of the RCT in relation to a heterogeneous communication problem like stammering, where each child's therapy is individualised according to their needs (for discussion of the issues see Pring, 2004). These limitations have led to the suggestion that appropriately designed and well-controlled single-subject studies that are replicated should be considered along with the RCT as a strong source of evidence (Kully & Langevin, 2005). In order to advance our research programme into Phase 3, we have carried out a multiple longitudinal single-subject study. There are a number of advantages to using this design with CWS. The use of repeated measures before the introduction of therapy allows the detection of any signs of pre-treatment recovery, and also enables observation of each child's individual variability, providing a more representative picture of a child's overall fluency skills (Ingham & Riley, 1998). The child's progress may then be measured against his normal variability in fluency, which eliminates the problem of withholding therapy. It is also argued that it is a more clinically relevant design, particularly for heterogeneous disorders, because it can be used within the context of regular clinical work (Pring, 2005).

Six children (aged 3:0–4:11 years) at risk of persistent stammering were monitored during a six-week baseline phase. This was followed by a six-week clinic-based therapy phase, a six-week home consolidation phase and a one-year post-therapy follow-up phase to enable the long-term impact of the therapy to be investigated (Millard *et al*, 2008). The frequency of stammering measures obtained during therapy and post-therapy were compared with the frequency and variability of stammering in the baseline phase. Like Jones *et al* (2005), we found that intervention with young CWS was beneficial. Four of the six children significantly reduced their stammering with both parents by the end of the *indirect* therapy phase (interaction and family strategies). One child significantly reduced the frequency of stammering with one parent only, while the remaining child made significant progress when the *direct* component of the Palin PCI programme (child strategies) was introduced. The four children who significantly reduced their stammering with both parents by the end of the therapy phase were discharged after the *indirect* component of Palin PCI therapy. These findings indicate that the *indirect* component of Palin PCI therapy may be effective on its own for some children, while more *direct* methods and ongoing therapy may be required for others. These results have been replicated with a further six children, all of whom significantly reduced their stammering within six months of receiving the *indirect* component of Palin PCI. This study also monitored, over the six-month period, the progress of four children who did not receive therapy. Of this group, only one child significantly reduced his stammering within the six months.

Phase 3:
Efficacy of Palin PCI (Millard et al, *2008)*

Analysis of parental ratings from all 12 children who received therapy showed that the positive changes in stammering frequency were supported by the parents' ratings of their child's stammer as being less severe. Parents rated themselves as being less concerned about the stammering and feeling more confident in their ability to manage it. The results demonstrated that Palin PCI therapy can reduce stammering in preschool children with six sessions of clinic-based therapy and six weeks of home consolidation.

The finding that 10 of the 12 participants were discharged having received only the *indirect* component of PCI therapy compares favourably with clinical outcome data reported in relation to other *indirect* approaches. Conture and Melnick (1999) reported discharge for 70 per cent of children after *indirect* therapy and Yaruss *et al* (2006) reported that 12 out of 17 children (approximately 70 per cent) achieved stammering frequency scores of three per cent or less at the end of therapy. We have therefore strengthened the support for the use of *indirect* methods with young children who stammer by replicating outcome across subjects within this study, and by considering the findings alongside previous studies. To date the majority of research into treatment effectiveness for young children who stammer has focused on one treatment approach, namely the Lidcombe Program (Jones *et al*, 2005; Lincoln & Onslow, 1997; Onslow *et al*, 2003; Onslow *et al*, 1994; Onslow *et al*, 1990). However, the findings of a pilot study have recently been reported by Franken *et al* (2005), who randomly assigned preschool children to either a Lidcombe Program (Onslow *et al*, 2003) or a Demands and Capacities Model treatment (see Adams, 1990; Gottwald & Starkweather, 1999; Starkweather *et al*, 1990). Preliminary findings suggest that there were no differences between the two treatment groups in terms of outcome. A larger study is currently being developed to investigate this further.

Having demonstrated that the Palin PCI programme is successful under optimal conditions, Phase 4 investigates its effectiveness when implemented in other settings with different subgroups of the clinical population of CWS. There are two single-subject studies that would constitute Phase 4 research in Palin PCI therapy (Crichton-Smith, 2002 ; Matthews *et al*, 1997), supporting the effectiveness of the programme when implemented in typical clinical environments.

Phase 5 research focuses on the issues of cost-effectiveness, client satisfaction and the effect of therapy on quality of life. Some of these are issues that are already being incorporated into much of our Phase 2 and Phase 3 research, as a result of the outcome measures we use.

Summary

The Robey and Schultz (1998) framework has helped to structure and prioritise research activities at the MPC. Research evidence is used to inform clinical decisions and contributes to evidence-based practice within the MPC. However, research evidence is not the only information considered. Expert experience and opinion is highly valued and feedback from our clients is regularly sought.

Initial Screening

2

Approximately 75 per cent of children who start to stammer will resolve the problem naturally (Kloth *et al*, 1999; Yairi & Ambrose, 1999). The challenge for us, as therapists, is to identify which children are at risk of persistence and to offer the most cost-effective and efficient form of intervention.

The initial screening will help the therapist select the appropriate care pathway for a child, based on whether he is at risk of persistence and therefore needs further assessment and intervention, or whether he is likely to recover and needs advice and monitoring.

The initial screening may take the form of a 20-minute appointment in the clinic, a postal questionnaire or a telephone call. The same information can be gathered using any of these methods.

If the referral indicates that the family's home language is other than English, an interpreter is booked for the clinic session. Alternatively, if we know that there is someone who can assist the parents in translating and completing the form at home, it is sent in the post.

Screening in the clinic

The child attends with one or both parents, and the therapist uses the 'Initial screening form' (see Appendix I) to gather information.

A suggested introduction:

'I have had a referral from... to have a look at your child's fluency. Did they talk to you about it? We have a slot for about 20 minutes and what I would like to do is ask you some questions about his speech. This will help me to work out what should be done next. I may need to bring you back to do a more detailed assessment or I may just give you some suggestions about what you can be doing to help.

When I talk about his speech I use the word 'stammering' to describe what is happening. What word have you been using? (if they say 'stutter' or 'dysfluency', say it all means the same thing).

It may be that ...'s speech is really fluent today - we know that they have good days and bad days so please don't worry - you can tell me what it is like when he is having trouble.'

Before the questions start, parents are asked to play with the child for a short time so that we can listen to the child's speech and note the type of stammering and any other speech and language issues. Given the variability of stammering in this age group, it is likely that the child will not stammer. We reassure parents that this is very common and we will not decide whether they need help based on this.

Questionnaire sent to parents

Alternatively, a copy of the 'Initial screening form' (see Appendix I) is sent to the parents, with an explanatory introduction, as suggested below.

'I have received a referral from... to assess your child's fluency. It would be helpful if you could complete this form as fully as possible as this will help me to work out what should be done next. When I have received your completed form I will send you an appointment to come to the clinic. At this point I may do a more detailed assessment or I may just give you some suggestions about what you can be doing to help.

Please note: *"stammering" means the same as "stuttering" or "dysfluency".'*

Telephone call

A further option is to obtain the screening information over the telephone, with the following explanation.

'I have received a referral from... to assess your child's fluency. I want to ask you some questions about him so that I can work out what should be done next. It will take about 20 minutes. When would be a good time for me to telephone you to do this?'

Before we ask the questions, we find out how the parent refers to the child's speech:

'When I talk about his speech I use the word "stammering" to describe what is happening. What word have you been using?' (if the parent says 'stutter' or 'dysfluency', say it all means the same thing).

Initial screening form

The 'Initial screening form' is used to gather the necessary information to identify the appropriate care pathway. Certain questions on the form are marked with a 'warning bell' (🔔), which denotes an area of risk for vulnerability to persistent stammering.

The form includes other questions, which do not indicate the level of vulnerability, but may be useful if the child is placed on the 'Advice & Monitoring' care pathway. We ask the parents to describe the stammering in detail and to rate its severity to provide baseline information to monitor the child's progress. We also enquire what seems to affect the child's fluency and how the parents instinctively respond to it. This informs any advice we may give on facilitating the child's fluency.

Planning the next step

The screening information is used to answer the following questions about the child's vulnerability to persistence, which will guide us to the appropriate management strategy:

- Is there is a family history of stammering?
- If so, did the stammering persist into adulthood?
- Are the parents worried about the child's speech?
- Has the child been stammering for more than 12 months?
- Has the stammering stayed the same or become worse?
- Does the child have any other speech or language difficulties?
- Has he had any other speech and language difficulties in the past?
- Are his language skills advanced?
- Is the child aware of his stammering?
- Is the child worried about his speech?

We don't need to hear the child stammering to decide whether he is at risk or what should be done

Although it is not possible to predict with 100 per cent accuracy the prognosis for any individual child, the responses to the questions will provide sufficient information to decide the appropriate care pathway:

- *No:* If the answers are 'No', then this child is likely to outgrow his fluency problem. He is placed on the 'Advice and Monitoring' care pathway, where the parents are given advice or specific tasks to facilitate the child's natural recovery, and then monitor his progress. These suggestions are given in Chapter 3.
- *Yes:* A 'Yes' to any of the questions suggests that the child may be vulnerable to persistent stammering and we make an appointment for

further assessment. The full assessment is used to gather more detailed information.

It will be helpful at this stage to agree with the child's parent or carer who will come to the case history session. Both parents are required to attend, or a single parent may bring a new partner or another main carer. If parents are no longer together, separate appointments for the case history may be offered.

In the discussion of risk factors in Chapter 1, we stated that no single factor is necessarily sufficient to predict the prognosis for a child. If there is only one risk factor for a child, a full assessment is still recommended, as this may reveal factors that may be affecting the child's fluency, for example a mismatch in language skills or other significant stresses in the family. However, if the child and the parents are not concerned about the speech, the child may be placed on the 'Advice and Monitoring' care pathway so that we may ensure that recovery is taking place.

Case study *Scott, aged three years*

Scott's mother reported that he had started to stammer a year ago and it had got steadily worse. He was prolonging and blocking, and sometimes giving up, saying, 'I can't say it.' His mother said she was really worried about it. Scott's father had stammered as a child and still did when he was under pressure. Scott's mother said that he had been an early talker and his language was better than other children of his age.

Warning bells

- *Scott aware and worried*
- *Stammer getting worse*
- *Mother worried*
- *Family history of persistence*
- *Advanced language skills*

Management *Full assessment*

Case study *Khaled, aged five years*

Khaled's mother reported that he had started to stammer about 18 months ago and it had fluctuated since then, not getting any better or worse. The stammer featured whole- and part-word repetitions and occasional prolongations, and Khaled did not seem to be aware of it. Khaled's maternal uncle had stammered as a child. Although he had grown out of the stammer, he had been teased about it at school, and Khaled's mother was really worried about Khaled experiencing the same thing. She said that the family spoke both Arabic and English at home and she felt that Khaled's language skills were fine, but his pronunciation of sounds had always been unclear.

Warning bells

- *Stammer not getting better*
- *Stammering for more than one year*
- *Mother worried*
- *Family history of stammering*
- *Speech sound difficulties*

Management *Full assessment*

Case study *Alfie, aged three and a half years*

Alfie started to stammer six months ago and a relative had told Alfie's mother to get him referred, although she said that she was not worried about it. She said that he was repeating words and parts of words, and sometimes prolonging sounds, but he was doing it less than he did at first and he had never shown any awareness of it. She felt that his other speech and language skills were as good as other children of his age.

Warning bells

- *There are no warning bells for this child*

Management *Advice and monitoring*

Advice and Monitoring

3

This care pathway is recommended for the child whose initial screening does not reveal a significant risk of persistent stammering, that is:

- There is no family history of stammering
- The parents are not worried about the child's speech
- The child has been stammering for less than 12 months
- The stammering is getting better
- The child's speech and language skills are within normal limits and not advanced
- The child has not had any other speech and language difficulties in the past
- The child is not aware of his stammering
- The child is not worried about his speech.

Information about stammering

Giving information about stammering and the risk factors can help parents understand how their child's fluency is developing and why the current stammering is likely to resolve. We want to reassure parents that they are right not to be worried about the child's speech (thus further reducing the likelihood of persistence).

Some suggestions are given below and this is outlined on the handout 'Information and advice for parents' (see Appendix II) that we give to the parents.

Information

Handout:
Information and advice for parents

- Fluency is a skill which gradually develops. Many children are hesitant in their speech as they learn new words, how to pronounce them and how to string words into sentences. When a child learns to walk, he may wobble, stumble and fall, especially in the early stages. Stumbling over sounds and words is a natural part of the process of learning to talk.
- Parents do not cause stammering.

- Four out of five young children who stammer will recover. There are a number of 'risk factors' which indicate which children are more likely to persist in stammering.
- The children who are most likely to recover from stammering are those who:
  - Are already showing signs of getting better
  - Don't have any relatives who stammer
  - Aren't aware or worried about their speech
  - Don't have any other problems with speaking
  - Don't have advanced language skills
  - Have been stammering for less than a year
  - Have parents who are not worried about the stammering.

Giving advice

During the initial screening the parents are asked what they feel affects their child's fluency and how they have been instinctively responding to it. In our experience many parents are aware of the influences on the child's speech – if he is excited or tired or trying to explain something complicated. They also often try to help the child by giving him advice when he stammers, for example 'take your time', 'calm down', 'take a breath'. This understanding and instinctive response is a useful starting point for giving the parents advice on how best to help their child's fluency.

- 'You say that his stammer is worse when he is excited, and you tell him to calm down. You are right that being calmer will help him to stammer less. Can you think of other ways, apart from telling him, in which you could help him to calm down?'
- 'You say that he stammers more when he is tired. Many parents say the same. Can you think of ways to help him not tire himself out so much or get more rest?'
- 'You say that his speech is worse when he is trying to explain something complicated. You are right, lots of children stammer more when they try to use sophisticated language. What do you think you could do to help him keep things fairly simple so that he is less likely to stammer?'
- 'When he stammers, you try to help him by telling him to breathe. How will stopping to take a breath help him not to stammer? Can you think of other ways you could help him to take a moment and keep calm?'

We can also give more general advice to parents on ways to help a child to be more fluent. However, it is important to remember that some of this advice involves the parents changing their style of interacting with the child, and we know that making these changes can be difficult. We therefore encourage parents to try out one or two of the following tips.

- When a child gives himself time, he can think and plan what he is trying to say and he can co-ordinate the movements involved in speaking. Many children rush to speak. A parent can set the pace for their child by trying to model pauses before they speak and by using an unhurried rate.
- We all ask questions, and when a child is asked a question, he is expected to respond. His ability to answer fluently will depend on how difficult the question is and how good his language skills are. Parents can help their child to answer more fluently by:
  - Avoiding questions which are too complicated for their child
  - Giving the child plenty of time to think of and give his reply
  - Avoiding asking another question before the child has had time to answer the first one.
- When we are in a group, we often overlap or interrupt each other. It can be harder for a child who stammers if he is rushing to finish what he wants to say before someone else butts in or if he is rushing to interrupt someone else. Parents can help their child by ensuring that everybody listens to each other and tries not to interrupt the speaker. The child will then feel able to take his time and this can help him to be more fluent. It's also important to remember to keep things fair – other family members should have their say, as well as the child who stammers.
- If parents are able to give their children some one-to-one 'quality' time, this may help the child who stammers as he has his parent's undivided attention and there is no need to rush. In a busy family lifestyle, parents may find it useful to have a brief (say, five minutes), regular slot with each child.

The various parents' handouts (see Appendices XIV – XVIII, XXI, XXII and XXIV – XXVII) may be useful for parents who are focusing on a particular way of helping their child to be more fluent.

Monitoring

We recommend review appointments at three months, six months and one year following the initial screening. This enables us to monitor that the child's fluency is continuing to improve. These reviews can take place over the telephone or in the clinic.

In these review sessions we ask parents to describe the stammering in the child's speech (see Chapter 2), as well as whether he seems to be growing aware of or worried about any stammering. We also ask parents to rate their own level of worry about the stammer on the 0 to 7 scale (see Chapter 2).

We then compare this information with the initial screening notes and decide with the parents if the stammering seems to be resolving. If the stammer seems to be getting worse or is causing anxiety, arrangements are made to do a full assessment.

If there are no concerns, we make a further review appointment, but reassure parents that they can contact us at any time should they become worried.

Case study *Alfie, aged three and a half years*

Alfie did not have any warning bells, that is:

- *There was no family history of stammering*
- *His mother was not worried about his speech*
- *He had been stammering for less than 12 months*
- *The stammering was getting better*
- *His speech and language skills were within normal limits and not advanced*
- *He had not had any other speech and language difficulties in the past*
- *He was not aware of or worried about his stammering.*

At the end of the initial screening, Alfie's mother was given information about stammering and a copy of the handout, with particular emphasis on the findings about his low vulnerability to persistence. She was reassured that his stammering was not a cause for concern, and told that if she felt that it was starting to get worse, or either of them were becoming concerned about it, she should contact us again. We arranged that we would telephone her three months later to check on Alfie's progress. Alfie was then monitored by telephone three, six and 12 months after the initial appointment. He had stopped stammering by the time of the six-month review and he was discharged after the 12-month review.

Note: *If, at any of these reviews, Alfie's mother had reported that the stammering was getting worse, or that either of them was concerned about it, a full assessment would have been arranged.*

4

Full Assessment

The overall aim of the full assessment is to generate information about factors which contribute to the onset and development of the child's stammer, as well as further details about the child's vulnerability to persistent stammering. Parents are central to the full assessment and provide valuable information about their child and his stammer within the context of the family.

Once the full assessment has been completed, the information is transferred onto a Summary Chart (see Appendix III). This assimilates the relevant information in order to present an explanation of the child's stammering to the parents. The Summary Chart also includes the possible range of strategies for the individualised treatment plan.

This chapter will include a description of each part of the full assessment procedure, including the recommended sequence, explanations and the use of forms which lead to the formulation and recommendations for therapy. We have included a flow chart (Figure 4.1 on page 44) which summarises the sequence of the full assessment and provides a reminder of which forms are to be filled in, and at which stage in the process.

The full assessment is undertaken when an initial screening has indicated that the child is vulnerable to persistent stammering. It comprises:

- parent–child interaction (PCI) video
- child assessment
- case history.

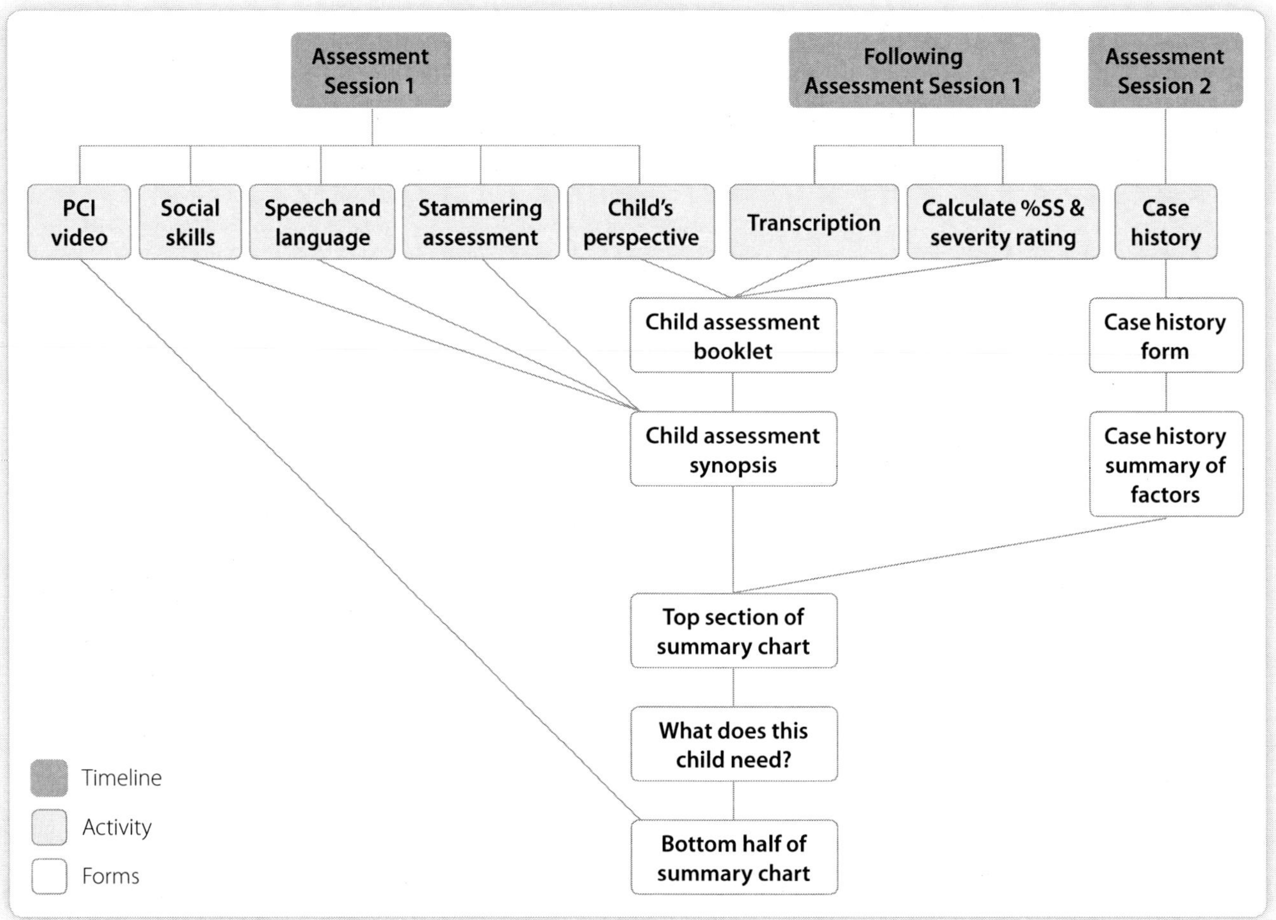

FIGURE 4.1 Full assessment: timeline, activities and forms to be completed

The full assessment

Assessment Session 1: PCI video and child assessment

Assessment Session 1 Equipment:
- *Video camera*
- *Play material*
- *Form boards or other similar activities*
- *Speech & language screening tools*
- *Tape recorder*
- *'What's Wrong?' pictures*
- *Child assessment booklet (see Appendix IV)*

The child attends with one or both parents for approximately one to one and a half hours.

After Session 1 the therapist will need one hour to complete the transcription and assessment analysis.

Assessment Session 2: case history, formulation and recommendations

The parents attend without the child for approximately two hours.

If the therapist is in a position to work collaboratively with another therapist, the whole assessment may take place on one occasion, with one therapist assessing the child while the other sees the parents. This provides a good opportunity for peer working and reflective practice.

PCI video

The child assessment session typically begins with the PCI video. This allows the child time to settle and become familiar with the clinic environment. Observation of the child playing with one or both of his parents can give us a useful indication of his level of fluency whilst interacting with his parents. We ask parents to complete a video consent form.

Setting up the initial PCI video

We want to reduce anxiety and encourage as natural and typical a playtime as possible. We give parents an explanation of the purpose of the video and what is required of them. We reassure parents that sometimes children are very quiet or very fluent during this video and that this does not matter. They will have time during the case history session to describe what happens in other situations.

An explanation:

'I would like to start by making a short video of each of you playing with your child. It is a useful way of settling him, and for me to have a snapshot of what he is like when he is playing with you, whom he knows well, rather than just seeing him with me, a stranger, It doesn't matter if he is very quiet; don't feel you have to get him to talk. Nor does it matter if he is very fluent, as we know that his fluency can vary from day to day.

I would like you to play with him for about five minutes, being as natural as you can be. I know that it is not the same as being at home but let's see if we can get a fairly typical picture of how things normally are.'

Typical play material:

- *Lego®*
- *Play mobile*
- *Train set*
- *Dolls house*

A choice of toys should be available, and we ask the child to choose what he would like to play with and which parent he would like to play with first. We make a video recording of each parent playing for about five minutes. It is often helpful to ask the parent who is not playing to sit outside or in a viewing room, if there is one. This is less distracting for the child.

The PCI analysis takes place after Assessment Session 1.

The child assessment

The child assessment takes place after the video recording of interaction and comprises the following:

- Screening of speech, language and social communication skills
- Assessment of stammering
- Child's perspective
- Completion of the 'Child assessment booklet' (see Appendix IV) and transfer of information to the Summary Chart (Appendix III).

Format of the child assessment

We have found that the following format usually enables us to gather all the necessary information within the constraints of the child's attention span:

- Settling activity at table, for example, form board
- Comprehension screening (requires non-verbal response at start)
- Expressive language and speech sound development screening
- Assessment of stammering
- Child's perspective.

The 'child's perspective' section is deliberately placed at the end of the assessment, as the child is likely to be more verbal at this stage; however, if there are concentration issues, we would ask the questions earlier in the session.

It may be necessary to intersperse the tasks above with other activities, for example, form boards or jigsaws, but they should be brief in order to make optimal use of the child's attention span. For some children, setting up a reward system, such as stickers, between tasks, also encourages their co-operation and helps them to maintain their concentration.

Screening of speech, language and social communication skills

A speech and language screen is essential to determine the linguistic factors that may be contributing to the current stammering

We routinely screen a child's speech, language and social communication skills to reveal the child's abilities and vulnerabilities.

Screening includes:

- Receptive language, including understanding of vocabulary and syntactic structures
- Expressive language, including vocabulary, syntax and use of language
- Word-finding ability
- Speech sound development
- Social communication skills.

It is then important to establish whether the child's:

- Speech, language and communication development are delayed or disordered
- Abilities are in line with each other, or if there is a mismatch between different areas, for example between receptive and expressive vocabulary or between expressive language and speech sound development
- Abilities are above the expected level for his chronological age.

The child's ability may fall within the average range on formal assessments, but there may be 'subclinical' or more subtle difficulties (see Chapter1).

Because therapists will already have a range of informal and formal speech and language assessments that they routinely use, we do not recommend any specific assessments for the child who stammers. Different tools will be used, depending on the age of the child. More in-depth speech and language assessment may be deemed necessary for some children, in which case further formal assessments may be used, again according to a therapist's preference.

We observe the child's social communication skills throughout the session.

Assessment of stammering

The aim of the assessment is to establish severity in terms of the frequency of the stammering and the types of stammering behaviours observed:

- Percentage of stammered syllables (%SS)
- Type of stammering behaviours
- Rate of speech.

Early stammering is variable from day to day, week to week and from situation to situation. There is a high chance that on the assessment occasion the child might present with little or no stammering. We will therefore check with the parents whether the sample obtained is representative of their child's stammering and gather further information about the child's fluency during the case history session. We also reassure parents that they will not be sent away with instructions 'not to worry' because their child did not stammer in the clinic.

A speech sample is audio- or video-recorded for fluency analysis. This sample can be taken during free play with the therapist or parents, but recording this can be difficult. Sitting at a table with picture material is usually easier. We recommend the LDA *'What's Wrong?'* pictures (LDA, 1988) as stimulus material as they are both entertaining and linguistically informative. We typically use about 10 pictures. If we are using an audiotape, we note any additional features, for example silent blocking and facial movements, as these will not be detectable from the recording.

This sample is later transcribed and analysed.

For further details on how to transcribe and annotate stammered speech and how to calculate the amount of stammering see the 'Assessment of stammering' (Appendix V).

The child's fluency is also observed during the rest of the assessment and in the PCI video.

From these observations and the analysis of the child's fluency, the following information is gathered:

- Percentage of stammered syllables, giving an indication of the amount of stammering on the assessment occasion.
- Types of stammering, including any tension, avoidance behaviours or concomitant movements.
- Rate of speech. We do not formally measure a child's rate of speech during the assessment but make a subjective judgement during different speaking tasks. We also consider the child's rate of speech in relation to their overall speech, language and co-ordination skills.

Clinical outcome measures:
- *%SS*
- *Yairi & Ambrose (2005) severity rating scale*

This information is summarised on the child assessment synopsis form (see Appendix IV) on the front of the 'Child assessment booklet'.

In addition, the Yairi and Ambrose (2005) severity rating scale may be used. This gives the stammering a numerical rating ranging from 0 = normal speech to 7 = very severe stuttering. Severity is based on the percentage of stammered syllables, the duration of the five longest episodes of stammering observed, as well as on the degree of tension and secondary behaviours present.

The child's perspective

We explore the child's awareness of his stammer through a simple line of questioning, starting with factual information about preschool or school and family. The child's responses to these questions are written on the 'Child assessment booklet' (see Appendix IV). This section includes a question about teasing. We ask the child whether he is being teased and if so what about.

Daniel, aged six years, said: 'It's hard for me to speak. It's like something's blocking the air. I have to take a big breath.'

Asking the child about his talking

Historically, it was strongly advised that stammering in a young child should be ignored and his attention not drawn to it. This was based on the fear that this would make the stammering worse. This is now discredited and therapists do not need to be anxious about asking the child direct questions about his stammering.

Kylie, aged four years, said: 'I go uh uh uh.'

Parents sometimes express concern about this aspect of the assessment, particularly when they have not told their child why they have brought him to the clinic. It is not unusual for parents to say that their child seems unaware of his stammering and has not shown any signs of concern. If necessary, we explain to parents why it is important to check whether their child is aware of his stammer and to reassure them that this will not make the problem worse. Many young children who experience stammering are aware of their speech problem.

We therefore ask the child direct questions about his speech, his feelings about it and whether he would like some help with it. This also gives us information about the child's level of insight and concern about his stammering as well as whether he has any strategies for managing it.

Kian, aged three years, said: 'I don't like having sticky words.'

Early signs of awareness may include a child looking away when stammering or generally appearing self-conscious when speaking. These kinds of reactions may be noticeable before a child directly comments on his speech.

It is usually clear when a child is not aware of any difficulty. He confidently reports that he is getting on fine with his talking and that it is always easy for him. We then do not ask the more specific questions about his speech.

Giving the child extra time to answer

The therapist will need to bear in mind that some children benefit from being given extra time to answer the questions about their speech. It may be the first time they have been given the opportunity to talk about their stammering and they may have to think about how to explain something so complicated.

Using the child's language

When a child does express awareness and can explain, we use his language in subsequent questions. For example, some children will talk about having a 'stammer', whereas others may say that their talking is 'hard' or 'wrong' or 'bumpy'. We would then ask: 'What happens when your talking is *wrong*?' or 'Would you like some help with your *bumpy talking*?'

Providing examples of stammering behaviours

Some children are aware of their stammering but find it difficult to describe. If a child says that he does have trouble talking, we might gently probe in the following way:

'Some of the children who come to see me find it hard to say their words and they say "My my my my name is…", do you ever do that? Or sometimes they say "My n-n-n-name is…", do you do that? Or sometimes they say "My naaame is…", do you do that? Or sometimes they say "My [block] name is…", do you do that?'

Some children are able to recognise their own speech patterns in these modelled examples, and this helps them to talk about their speech further. In our experience, children who are unaware of their stammering, or who do not wish to talk about it, will just say, '*No, I don't do that.*'

Child assessment synopsis and Summary Chart completed

Once the child has left the session we analyse the speech and language assessments, and transcribe and analyse the speech sample collected for the assessment of stammering. We summarise these assessment findings in the 'Child assessment booklet', together with comments about the child's social communication skills. This information is then transferred to the top section of the Summary Chart, as shown on p.51.

> ***Case study*** *Scott, aged three years*
>
> Child assessment
>
> *Scott was highly co-operative and concentrated well. He took turns in the conversation, but his turns were lengthy. He used eye contact except during moments of blocking, when he would look away. He seemed anxious to perform well, often asking* 'Was that right?' *He wanted to finish tasks quickly and carefully lined up the* 'What's Wrong?' *cards in a straight row.*
>
> *Scott presented with a moderate stammer, featuring whole- and part-word repetitions with up to three repetitions, prolongations for up to three seconds and blocking. He stammered on 9.8 per cent of syllables spoken. When asked how he was getting on with his talking he said* 'I can't say my words.'
>
> *His receptive and expressive language skills were sophisticated, at over a five-year level. He tended to talk at length and used a rapid rate of speech.*

See Appendix VI for Scott's completed child assessment synopsis

> ***Case study*** *Khaled, aged five years*
>
> Child assessment
>
> *Khaled was initially quiet but settled quickly. He co-operated well and his use of eye contact and turn-taking skills were appropriate.*
>
> *Khaled presented with a mild stammer, featuring whole- and part-word repetitions and one prolongation. He stammered on six per cent of syllables spoken and there was no associated tension. He seemed to talk using a rapid rate of speech. When asked about how he was getting on with his talking, he said it was 'OK.'*
>
> *Screening of his receptive and expressive language skills showed that these were developing normally, but his speech sound system featured delayed phonological development, which made it difficult to understand him at times.*

See Appendix VII for Khaled's completed child assessment synopsis

The top section of the Summary Chart (Figure 4.2) represents the child's profile of abilities and underlying vulnerabilities.

Information from the child assessment (and later the case history) is used to begin to identify significant aspects of the child's profile of abilities and vulnerabilities which may contribute to his stammer.

A tick is placed in the column next to each relevant aspect from the assessment.

Stammering & Social Communication Skills			
% ss *Parent rating*		Child's awareness/concern	
Type of stammering *WWR PWR Prol. Blocking*		Talking at length/turn-taking	
Time since onset *< 6mths <12mths >12mths*		Reduced eye contact	
Pattern of change *Better Same Worse*		Reduced concentration	
Parents' levels of concern		**Linguistic**	
		History of delayed speech/language development	
Physiological		Reduced receptive skills	
Family history of stammering		Reduced expressive skills	
Co-ordination		Word finding difficulty	
Tiredness		Speech sound difficulty	
Birth history		Advanced language skills	
Health		Mismatch within/between speech/language skills	
Rapid bursts/rate of speech		Managing two languages	
Psychological		**Environmental**	
Reduced confidence		Turn-taking in family	
High standards		Behaviour management	
Increased sensitivity		Routines	
Anxious/worrier		Openness about stammering	
Difficulties coping with change		Preschool/school issues	
Reaction to stammering		Pace of life	

FIGURE 4.2 Top section of the Summary Chart

What does this child need?

The middle section of the Summary Chart (Figure 4.3) is then completed. We consider what the child needs in order to be more fluent: this will outline the general aims of the therapy programme for that child, for example:

- To give himself more time and be given time by others
- To develop his expressive language
- To further develop his confidence.

What does this child need?
1
2
3

FIGURE 4.3 Middle section of the Summary Chart

Case study *Scott, aged three years*

Scott's needs:

1. *To take the pressure off himself by giving himself more time.*
2. *To use shorter, simpler utterances.*
3. *Not to set himself standards that are too high.*

Case study *Khaled, aged five years*

Khaled's needs:

1. *To give himself time to plan and execute speech.*
2. *To develop his speech sound system.*

Analysis of PCI Video

Included in the bottom section of the Summary Chart is a list of interaction strategies (Figure 4.4) which guide us when analysing the PCI video. This preliminary analysis of the PCI video is carried out using the information gained from the child assessment.

INTERACTION STRATEGIES	Helpful	Evidence of		Potential target	
		Mother	Father	Mother	Father
Following child's lead in play					
Letting child solve problems					
More comments than questions					
Complexity of questions at child's level					
Language is appropriate to child's level					
Language is semantically contingent on child's focus					
Repetition, expansion, rephrasing					
Time to initiate, respond, finish					
Rate of input when compared with child's rate					
Use of pausing					
Using eye contact, position, touch, humour and/or surprise					
Praise and encouragement					

FIGURE 4.4 Interaction strategies on the Summary Chart

We consider the patterns of interaction between each parent and the child from two perspectives:

- The child's profile of speech, language and communication abilities and underlying vulnerabilities
- Fluency-facilitating strategies or, if relevant, language-facilitating strategies already used by the parent.

There are no standard interaction strategies recommended for all parents and not all of the facilitative styles listed will be appropriate for a parent to use. Certain strategies are only appropriate if the child has a specific difficulty, for example we may need to think about the length and complexity of a parent's input for a child with reduced language skills.

Helpful

The column marked 'Helpful' is ticked to begin with, to indicate to the therapist which interaction strategies would be appropriate given the child's profile of abilities and vulnerabilities.

Evidence of

Once we have identified which interaction strategies might be helpful for the child's fluency, the Summary Chart may then be used to evaluate each parent's use of the relevant strategies, by ticking the 'Evidence of' column. This is done by watching the video recording of each parent playing with the child. If there are two parents, we record their use of interaction strategies individually in the column marked 'Mother' or 'Father'.

We look for examples of a parent using any of the strategies that we have selected as being potentially 'Helpful'. The relevant box in the 'Evidence of' column is then ticked to indicate that the parent is already using that strategy.

Potential target

If we feel that it would be helpful for the parent to use a strategy more often, we identify it as a potential target for therapy by ticking the 'Potential target' column.

This preliminary analysis of the PCI video provides us with information for the formulation (see Chapter 5) and guides our decision-making process when selecting therapy. We may return to the PCI video before the formulation to include the information gained from the case history session. For example, during the case history parents may have described their child as being independent and said that he likes to do things for himself. We may therefore focus on the times when parents follow his lead in play.

(a)

INTERACTION STRATEGIES	Helpful	Evidence of		Potential target	
		Mother	Father	Mother	Father
Following child's lead in play	✓	✓	✓	✓	
Letting child solve problems					
More comments than questions	✓	✓	✓		
Complexity of questions at child's level	✓	✓	✓		
Language is appropriate to child's level	✓	✓	✓		
Language is semantically contingent on child's focus	✓	✓	✓		
Repetition, expansion, rephrasing					
Time to initiate, respond, finish	✓	✓	✓	✓	✓
Rate of input when compared with child's rate	✓	✓	✓		✓
Use of pausing	✓	✓	✓	✓	✓
Using eye contact, position, touch, humour and/or surprise	✓	✓	✓	✓	
Praise and encouragement	✓	✓	✓		

(b)

INTERACTION STRATEGIES	Helpful	Evidence of		Potential target	
		Mother	Father	Mother	Father
Following child's lead in play	✓	✓		✓	
Letting child solve problems	✓				
More comments than questions	✓	✓			
Complexity of questions at child's level	✓	✓			
Language is appropriate to child's level	✓	✓			
Language is semantically contingent on child's focus	✓	✓			
Repetition, expansion, rephrasing	✓	✓		✓	
Time to initiate, respond, finish	✓	✓		✓	
Rate of input when compared with child's rate	✓	✓		✓	
Use of pausing	✓	✓		✓	
Using eye contact, position, touch, humour and/or surprise	✓	✓			
Praise and encouragement	✓	✓			

FIGURE 4.5 Interaction strategies for (a) Scott (aged three) and (b) Khaled (aged five)

The case history

The case history

- *Involves both parents or main carers*
- *Efficient and cost-effective*
- *Supportive for the child*
- *Assists transfer of skills into the family*
- *Shared responsibility for change*
- *Shared understanding*

We require both parents (where appropriate) or the child's main carers to attend the case history session. Clearly, there are circumstances where this is inappropriate, for example a single parent who is not in contact with the other parent. Parents who have separated may be able to attend together to help the child, but this may not be appropriate if the relationship is not amicable. We have often invited such parents to attend on separate occasions. Some parents are away from home because of work commitments (eg, the armed forces, oil industry) or personal circumstances (eg, refugee families).

Parents are asked to attend without any children. This enables them to be more open about their child's stammer and their feelings about it. In addition, it allows them to discuss any other concerns they have about the child or any difficulties within the family which they feel may be affecting the child's stammer.

Taking the case history

The case history consists of a series of questions aimed at finding out about the child and his stammer within the context of the family. This enables us to identify which factors may have contributed to its onset and development, and it provides further information about the child's level of vulnerability to persistent stammering. The child's parents are the obvious source of this information, but they may worry that they are to blame or are doing something wrong. It is therefore important to allay any such worries or fears from the outset. We typically do this at the beginning of the session by saying something like the following.

'Stammering is a complex problem and there has been a great deal of research into what causes it. We know, and the research confirms, that parents do not cause stammering. You know your child better than anyone and that is why I need your help with the assessment. The questions I ask you are designed to help me understand more about your child and his stammering. The questions do not have right answers or wrong answers (and the two of you may have different opinions).

When we have finished the case history, I will put the information you have given me together with the information from the child assessment. I will then explain to you which factors may be contributing to the stammering and what we need to do about it. I will also give you some general information about stammering and answer any questions you may have.'

The case history form is set out in Appendix VIII. It is divided into the following sections:

- Biographical details
- Presenting problem
- Communication
- Health and development
- Eating and sleeping
- Personality
- Child's relationships
- Family history
- Family relationships
- Schooling
- Behaviour management
- Developmental history.

We have tried to set out the questions using plain English. It may be necessary to reword some questions if clarification is required. For example:

- *'Is he sensitive?'* (Is he very aware of other people's feelings? Does he worry when other people are upset?)
- *'Does he have difficulties with co-ordination?'* (Does he seem clumsy? Can he ride a bike, catch a ball, do up his buttons?)

Some of the questions address areas which may have already been covered either during the initial screening or the child assessment. However, it is still important to ask the parents all the questions for a number of reasons.

- The information gleaned from the initial screening and child assessment may be an incomplete picture.
- Although some of the questions are identical to those used in the initial screening, in the interim the child's stammering and the parents' reactions may have changed, or they may have noticed other features.
- It is generally more meaningful for the parents if they have noticed something about their child, rather than if we describe it to them.

The parents' responses are written on the case history form as we go along. We also highlight on the form key information which seems to be relevant in understanding the child's stammering.

Confidentiality

Each speech and language therapy service will have its own standard phrases, which are used to explain confidentiality to parents and when and how that confidentiality may be broken. Typically:

'The assessment is confidential to the Centre, but should I become concerned about your child's welfare at any time, as a professional, I am obliged to pass on information to other agencies, as needed.'

Parent–therapist relationship

Although the therapist has already met one or both parents during the child assessment, the case history session marks the beginning of a therapeutic relationship between the parents and the therapist, and this will be important for the ultimate success of any therapy which may later be needed. The therapist will demonstrate her empathy with the parents' feelings, hopes and concerns, and will aim to develop a relationship based on mutual trust and understanding.

The case history form (see Appendix VIII) consists of both direct and open-ended questions, and parents are encouraged to describe their concerns in their own words. Eliciting information from parents involves the use of core counselling skills: specifically, asking questions, active listening, accepting, reflecting and summarising.

Understanding the rationale

It is important to understand the rationale of each question on the case history form. In our experience, therapists are more confident about asking questions once they have understood the rationale behind them. Although parents are usually happy to respond to all the questions asked, we need to be ready to explain why we ask each question.

Noticing the words parents use

A note is made of the parents' terms of reference so that we can quote them directly during the formulation. This is because parents' own words are more meaningful to them than ones chosen by us. For example if the parents report that the child sometimes has trouble thinking of the word he wants to say, this might have more impact than informing them that he has a word-finding problem.

Structure of the interview

The interview is structured in order to minimise the opportunities to become side-tracked and to make sure that we cover all the factors. Parents are often keen to tell us as much as possible about their child's fluency; however, this may result in us moving back and forth from one page of the interview to the next in order to keep a record of their comments. The danger of doing this is that questions may be missed. Although parents are encouraged to give us as much information as possible, we may ask them to hold back some information if questions related to that topic will be asked later. For example, 'That is important, if we could just finish ..., we'll come back to that later.'

Waiting until the formulation before giving advice and information

Sometimes parents are keen to be given information or advice about their child's stammering during the interview. They may ask direct questions about the cause of their child's stammering: whether he will grow out of it and how they should respond and so on. Instead of answering questions during the case history, we reassure parents that there will be time at the end of the session to come back to any questions. Advice given to parents will be more accurate once the assessment has been completed and parents may also be more receptive to recommendations once a complete understanding of their child has been obtained.

Presenting problem

- 'Are there any other problems apart from the stammering that you are worried about?'
- 'If so, which is your main concern at the moment?'

We begin the interview by asking the parents whether their child has any other problems apart from the stammering. For example, health or behaviour problems, delays in other areas of their development and so forth. When other concerns are expressed, it is important to establish which problem the parents are most concerned about. This helps us to understand the context of the child's stammering problem and how it fits in with the family's other priorities.

Description of stammer

- 'What does he do when he stammers?'

As we explained earlier, it is important to gather information about the child's stammering directly from parents, as the child's level of fluency during the child assessment may not be representative of his typical speech. We encourage parents to give as full a description as possible of their child's fluency. Some parents are able to describe accurately the features of their child's stammer, whilst others will benefit from being asked more specific questions and given examples of different types of stammering, for example, 'Does he repeat whole words eg, *but but but*?' 'Repeat parts of words eg, *b-b-but*?' 'Stretch sounds eg, *mmmmum*?' 'Get stuck on a sound and nothing comes out?' 'Does he do anything else with his face or body when he stammers?' 'Does he do anything to try to hide it?'

Child's awareness and response to his stammer

- 'Does he avoid words?', 'Situations?', 'Does he ever give up saying something?'
- 'Do you think he is aware of it?', 'Concerned about it?', 'What gives that impression?'
- 'Do you think his stammer affects his confidence?'

It is important to establish whether the child is aware of the problem and what impact it is having on his communication and confidence. Some children are very aware of their stammer from an early age and have started opting out of speaking because of it. Clinical experience indicates that when a child is aware of the problem, and is already reacting to it, the stammering is typically a more significant problem.

Strategies for managing stammer

- 'Does he seem to have any strategies for managing his stammer?'

A child may already be attempting different strategies for managing his stammer. It is important to know what these strategies are, and whether they are helpful. Parents may have taught the child ways of managing the stammer or they may have learnt some strategies during previous speech and language therapy sessions.

Onset of stammer

- 'When did he start stammering?'
- 'Was there anything in particular going on in his life at that time?'(eg, changes in preschool, school, birth of a sibling, family moving, other family changes or events?)
- 'Did it start gradually or suddenly?'
- 'Has it changed since then? In what way?'

We want to know how long a child has already been stammering. Parents may find it difficult to give a time of onset, especially if it was gradual, but asking them to tie it in with events in the child's life, such as starting preschool, family holiday, birth of a sibling, moving house may help them to be more specific. The onset of stammering may be sudden, and it can be severe right from the beginning, which can cause parents a great deal of concern, particularly when their child was developing fluency normally before this.

Times when stammer is better or worse

- 'When is the stammering worse?' or 'When does it happen the most?'
- 'When is the stammering better?' or 'When does it happen the least?'

Some parents will have a clear idea about when their child's stammering is better and when it is worse. They often report that it is worse when he is excited, or in a hurry to explain something complicated. Other parents report that they have not noticed any particular pattern to their child's stammering.

Talking about the stammering with the child

- 'Do you talk about the stammering with your child?'

Some parents are already very open about the child's stammer and are able to discuss it in a matter of fact way. Others are concerned about discussing it in case they make it worse. As before, we help parents to understand that it is fine to talk openly about the stammer.

Parents' responses:
'I know it helps when I give him some one-to-one time'
'I do talk a bit fast so I try and slow down when I'm talking to her'
'I do sometimes say, "Oh dear that was a bit hard to say"'

How parents respond to the stammer

- 'What do you do or say when your child stammers?'

We ask each parent what they, and any siblings, do to help their child when he stammers. This will give us an indication of the kind of feedback the child is getting. Each parent may have a different way of responding to the child's stammer.

What seems to help him most?

Parents often have instincts about what is most helpful for their child and we elicit this information to use and develop in therapy. Typically, parents' responses include not having to rush, having time to think about what he is trying to say, not being interrupted and having individual time with his parents.

Parents' rating of severity and their level of concern

- 'On a scale of 0–7, where 0 is normal and 7 is very severe, how severe is his stammer?'

Mother	0	1	2	3	4	5	6	7
Father	0	1	2	3	4	5	6	7

- 'On a scale of 0–7, where 0 is not at all worried and 7 is extremely worried, where are you now?'

Mother	0	1	2	3	4	5	6	7
Father	0	1	2	3	4	5	6	7

Clinical outcome measures
Parents' rating of:
- *Severity*
- *Level of concern*

We ask parents to rate the severity of their child's stammering, using the Yairi and Ambrose (2005) eight-point severity rating scale. Using the same scale, we also ask parents to rate their level of concern about it. This gives us an initial measure of their view of the problem. It is not unusual for each parent to give a different rating of severity and their level of concern about it. We can repeat these ratings after therapy to establish any changes in parents' rating of the problem. Parental level of concern is sometimes a key factor in deciding what recommendations will be appropriate.

Previous therapy and expectations

- 'Has your child had therapy before?'
- 'What happened?'
- 'What are you hoping for today?'

We want to know if parents have already received some speech and language therapy support or any other help. This will give us an insight into what parents have already gained from therapy and what they already know about what helps their child's fluency. It is also important to establish parents' expectations of therapy. This may reveal unrealistic hopes, which will need to be addressed at the end of the case history in light of the child's profile of vulnerability to persistent stammering.

Communication

- 'Does he have any other problems with communication, speech, or language?'
- 'Does he speak as well as other children of the same age?'
- 'Does he speak clearly?'
- 'What is his rate of speech like?'

Although we will have gathered information about the child's speech, language and communication abilities during the child assessment, it is useful to hear the parents' perspective. We also ask for their views on their child's rate of talking. This is clearly a very subjective measure, but parents often have an instinct that the child is sometimes going too fast for himself, especially when he is excited.

Bi- or multilingual

- 'Does your child speak more than one language?'
- 'If so, what language is spoken at home?'
- 'Which does he use the most?'
- 'Are there any differences in his stammering in the languages?'

For children from bilingual or multilingual backgrounds, it is important to establish which other languages are spoken in the home and by the child. Parents often feel that their child's fluency is better in one language than the other.

Health and development

Health

- 'How is your child's general health?'

Parents may sometimes be worried about their child's health, which may be a greater concern at the time of the assessment. If health concerns are identified, we need to understand the impact these might be having on the child and the family. Parents may feel that the child's stammering seems to be worse when he is unwell.

Hearing

- 'Have you ever had concerns about his hearing?'
- 'Has his hearing ever been tested?'

Some of the questions asked during the case history are the same as those routinely asked during any initial speech and language therapy assessment. We ask parents about their child's hearing and the results of any hearing tests. Typically, hearing tests have already been carried out, but if the parents are expressing concern and hearing has not been tested, we recommend a referral.

Concentration

- 'What is his concentration like?'
- 'Is he fidgety or restless?'

We ask parents to comment on their child's concentration. When parents feel that their child does not concentrate as well as other children of his age, it is also helpful to find out if there are concerns about his concentration at preschool or school. The child's concentration will also have been observed during the child assessment.

Co-ordination

- 'What is his co-ordination like?'

Although the child's co-ordination will have been observed during the child assessment, it is useful to hear the parents' perspective. If parents raise specific concerns about the child's gross or fine motor skills, or difficulties are identified during the child assessment, we may need to refer the child to physiotherapy or occupational therapy for assessment and ongoing support.

Eating and sleeping

Eating

- 'Are there any problems with eating or mealtimes?'
- 'If so, what?'
- 'How do you manage the problem?'
- 'Do you always agree on how to manage it?'
- ' What helps most?'

We ask about the child's eating habits for two reasons: first, if the child has any physical difficulties with chewing and swallowing or if he is a very messy eater, this may indicate an oro-motor problem. Second, eating and mealtimes can become an area of conflict between a parent and child which may be affecting the family as a whole.

Sleeping

- 'What about sleeping?'
- 'What time does he go to bed?'
- 'When does he wake?'
- 'Does he sleep through the night?'
- 'Does he stay in his own bed?'
- 'Do you think he gets enough sleep?'

Many parents report that their child is more fluent when he is well-rested. We need specific information about bedtime routines to understand whether the child is getting enough sleep. Parents may report that they are finding bedtimes difficult to manage, for example the child not wanting to go to bed or not staying in his own bed. Parents may be very tired themselves owing to their child's sleeping routine and, as a result, are finding it harder to manage the child during the day.

Personality

- 'How would you describe your child's personality?'
- 'Would you say that he is sensitive, or not particularly?' (Examples)
- 'How does he react if he gets something wrong or makes a mistake?' (Examples)
- 'Does he like to please?'
- 'Does he worry, or not particularly?' (Examples)
- 'Does he get upset easily, or not particularly?' (Examples)
- 'Who does he take after?'
- 'Does he have a temper?'
- 'If so, how does he show his temper?'

- 'Which situations trigger it?'
- 'Is his temper an issue at school?'
- 'How do you deal with it?'
- 'How does he cope with changes, new places and experiences?'
- 'Is he a child who likes routine?'
- 'How is he doing in terms of developing independence?'

A child's temperament may play a role in how he reacts to and manages the stammering in his speech. A child who is a born worrier or highly sensitive or has high standards may be more likely to notice and react to the stammer. He may respond to moments of difficulty and put himself under greater pressure.

We start by asking the parents to describe their child's personality in their own words. This is then followed by a list of prompts to gather more detailed information about the child's personality. For example, 'Would you say that he is sensitive, or not particularly?' 'Is he a worrier, or not particularly?' 'Does he like to please?' In our experience, parents often describe their child as being highly sensitive, a worrier or a perfectionist.

We include a question about temper tantrums: what situations typically prompt them and how parents are already managing such situations.

We also ask about routines because our experience has shown that some children thrive in the predictability and safety of a routine, and flounder when the routine is not in place. It may be that the stammering becomes more marked when there is less routine, such as during holidays. Some children's need for routine may extend to 'ritualistic' behaviour, for example, insisting on a rigid pattern of events or layout of possessions. If this behaviour is extreme, it may be an indicator of an underlying anxiety or other problem, so further investigation or help may be necessary.

Child's relationships

- 'How does your child get on with other children?'
- 'Does he have friends?'
- 'Does he see them outside preschool or school?'
- 'Is he ever teased or bullied?'
- 'Does he get into fights?'

The child's relationships with other children and any siblings give further insight into his personality and social interaction skills. It is also important to establish whether a child's stammering is interfering with his relationships. If the child is being teased or bullied this may affect his awareness and anxiety about the stammering. It is useful to find out how such incidents are being handled by the child, parents or the preschool or school.

- Names and ages of brothers and sisters
- 'How do they get on?'

Rivalry is common among siblings and may not be a cause for concern. However, it is helpful to determine if a child is putting himself (and thereby his fluency) under pressure by competing with an older sibling, or by trying to stay one step ahead of a bright younger sibling.

How does he manage during family conversations?

We will have made observations about the child's turn-taking during the child assessment and also noted how the parents manage turns between them during the case history. It is also useful to ask parents about the turn-taking patterns within the home when all the family is together. We want to know whether family members take turns to talk, or whether there is competition for talking time, or a tendency to interrupt each other.

Family history

- 'Have parents or other family members ever stammered?'
- 'If so, do they still stammer?'
- 'Have they had therapy?'
- 'If so, what was the outcome?'

These questions were asked at the initial screening and are repeated now, as parents who did not previously know about any family history may, by now, have found out some details. If there is a family history, it is important to find out whether or not family members have recovered or have persistent stammering. Sometimes the information is not available, for example if the child is adopted and such details are not known about the birth parents, or if parents have separated and this information is not available about a parent or extended family members.

During the interview a parent may say that he stammers or used to stammer when he was younger. This is of interest because a parent's experience and attitude to his own stammering may be having an impact on how he feels and manages his child's stammering. For example:

- A parent who has never talked about their own stammer may find it difficult to understand the rationale of being open and acknowledging their child's stammering. Alternatively, a parent may find it perfectly natural to talk to their child about his stammer even though they do not openly discuss their own stammer.

- Information about a parent's own experience of speech and language therapy is also important and may influence their expectations of therapy for their child.
- A parent who stammers may feel guilty as they might feel they have caused the child's stammering.
- If a parent has recovered from stammering they may feel that their child will also grow out of it, which may affect their attitude to therapy.

We may observe that a parent is not very fluent; however, they do not describe themselves as having a stammer. As there is no precise point on the fluency continuum at which stammering is 'diagnosed', the parent may just view himself as a hesitant speaker, or may have no awareness of his level of fluency. It is not our role to label people so we would just make a note of the parent's level of fluency in such a case.

Family relationships

- 'How long have you been together/married?'
- 'Have you had any separations?'
- 'If so, can you tell me a bit about what happened?'
- 'How did your child cope with the changes?'
- 'How would you say you get on as a couple?'

We ask parents about their relationship in order to find out if there are disruptions or conflicts in the home which may be affecting the child. Therapists often express concern about asking these questions. Our experience is that once therapists have understood the rationale behind them they are able to ask them confidently.

Some parents may link their child starting to stammer with a period of time when their relationship was difficult or there was a relationship breakdown. If this is the case it will be important to reassure them that this will not have caused their child to start to stammer. It may be that their child was vulnerable to fluency breakdown from the outset, for example owing to a family history of stammering. The onset of the stammering happened to coincide with this period in their life. If there are difficulties in the parents' relationship, this may be important in deciding when we start therapy. It may be appropriate to recommend relationship counselling.

One-parent families

- 'What contact does your child have with the other parent?'
- 'Who has full parental responsibility?'
- 'Have either of you started new relationships?'

- 'How does your child feel about these issues at the moment?'
- 'Do you have any concerns?'

For one-parent families, we gather information about the child's contact and relationship with the other parent. We establish who has parental responsibility and whether there are issues around custody and access. In addition, it is important to establish whether either parent has started a new relationship and any impact of this on the child who stammers.

Schooling

- 'How did your child first cope with going to preschool or school?'
- 'Do you have any concerns about his schooling?'
- 'Are any changes planned?'
- 'What feedback do you get from staff?'
- 'Do you think he needs extra support?'
- 'Does he have an Individual Education Plan?'
- 'Are the teachers concerned about his stammer?'
- 'What do his teachers do when he stammers?'

The child's preschool or school environment may have some impact on his fluency, so we need to establish how well he copes with the social, educational and behavioural demands. If a child is struggling to cope with the academic expectations of early school, his fluency may also be under some pressure.

We need to know about the teachers' management of the child's stammering. Preschool staff and teachers may have experience of early stammering, and expect that the child will outgrow the problem. It is helpful to find out if the parents have any concerns about the school's handling of their child's difficulty. It may be appropriate for us to contact the preschool or school directly to discuss the child's stammer (see Chapter 8).

Behaviour management

- 'What do you do when he is naughty or needs discipline?'
- 'Do you both manage this in the same way?'
- 'Are you consistent?'
- 'How does he react?'
- 'Is there anything that is difficult to manage at the moment?'

Parents will have different styles and methods of managing a child's behaviour, influenced by their own experiences as a child, as well as cultural norms and expectations. We do not stand in judgement of their methods (provided they are legal). It is helpful to learn about their systems and to establish whether they are having difficulties in this area. Parents may be concerned that their management of the child's behaviour might make the stammering worse. Some parents feel they have become locked into a negative pattern of behaviour with their child which they feel is unhelpful, for example at bedtime. If there are frequent behaviour management issues in the family home, this may be affecting a child's fluency. Our therapy may therefore include supporting the parents with managing their child's behaviour or we may need to make an onward referral to Child and Adolescent Mental Health Services (CAMHS).

Developmental history

- 'Were there any complications during the pregnancy or birth?'
- 'Was he a full-term baby?'
- 'What was his birth weight?'
- 'Were there any difficulties with feeding or other complications?'
- 'Were there any early difficulties during infancy?'
- 'When did he start to walk?'
- 'When did he say his first words?'
- 'When did he say his first simple sentences?'
- 'When did he come out of nappies?'
- 'Were there any developmental problems?'

This section of the case history consists of the standard questions included in a speech and language therapy case history form.

We usually conclude the case history by asking parents if there is anything else we should know about their child that hasn't already been discussed or if there are any other concerns that have not been mentioned.

> ***Case study*** *Scott, aged three years*
>
> *At the case history Scott's parents described the same stammering behaviours as those noted at the child assessment. They also reported that he was giving up more often, sometimes saying 'I can't say it.' They said that they did not know what to say when he said this, as they didn't want to make it worse by sounding worried about it. They reported that he clenched his fists when his stammer was most severe. Scott had started to stammer at the age of two. He had been stammering for 14 months and they felt that it was still getting worse. They noticed that he was more fluent when he was calm and when he was talking in a one-to-one setting. He was worse when he was giving complicated explanations, when he was excited or when he was competing to speak with his twin sister. They thought that what seemed to help him was*

when he 'kept it short and sweet,' when he had plenty of time and when he was not trying to watch the television at the same time as speaking. His mother rated his stammering severity as seven and his father rated it as six. They both rated their own level of concern as six.

Both parents felt that Scott's language skills were very good and that he often tried to talk very fast, especially when his sister was around. They reported no problems with his health or eating and sleeping.

They described Scott as a kind and loving boy who was very bright and wanted to do well. He was very aware of other people's feelings and liked to please. He was very competitive with his sister and he was careful and tidy. They felt that he tended to worry about things but he often kept his worries to himself. They said that he was a confident child but they were concerned that his confidence might decrease as he became more aware of his stammering.

Scott's parents reported that, in addition to the family history of Scott's father's stammering, they had also discovered that his grandfather and great-uncle stammered as adults. Scott's mother also said that she was dyslexic.

Scott's parents described their own relationship as being 'pretty normal.' They had no concerns about his preschool. They did not feel there were any difficulties with managing his behaviour.

Scott's birth and developmental history was normal.

Case study *Khaled, aged five years*

Khaled's mother, who was a single parent, said that when he stammered Khaled repeated parts of words and whole words and that he prolonged sounds. She said that he didn't seem to notice his stammering and it was not stopping him from doing anything. Khaled had started to stammer when he began to use longer sentences, when he was about three and a half. He was worse when he was tired, frustrated or in a hurry. She thought that he seemed to be helped when 'he took it slowly' and she usually told him to slow down when he started to stammer. She rated the severity of Khaled's stammering at three on the rating scale and she rated her own level of concern as being six.

She felt that his language was about the same as other children of his age, but his speech had never been very clear and other people often did not understand him, although she usually did. The family spoke Arabic and English at home but she said whilst he understood Arabic well, Khaled seemed to prefer to speak in English since going to school.

Khaled's mother said that he was a messy eater and she found it very difficult to get him to go to sleep at night. She felt that he was often overtired and so was she.

She described Khaled as a happy boy who wanted to have his own way, but he was not sensitive and did not worry about things. He had a bit of a temper, especially when he could not do or have what he wanted. She felt that he was fairly confident at home but she was not sure he was the same at preschool with other children. Khaled had a seven-year-old brother who he would play and fight with, and his mother thought that this was 'pretty normal'.

Khaled's mother talked about her own younger brother, who stammered as a child and was teased about this at school, often coming to her in the playground in tears. She said that this made her feel very worried that Khaled might face the same thing at school. Her brother had stopped stammering by the time he went to secondary school. Khaled's mother had been on her own since he was six months old and there was no contact with his father as he was living in Algeria. Some members of the extended family lived nearby and gave her lots of help.

She described her difficulties managing Khaled's behaviour when he couldn't get his own way. He would get so frustrated and often this would make him stammer more. She said that she tried to be firm but sometimes she gave in. She found it really difficult when he would not go to bed at night.

Preparing the formulation

When we have completed the case history, there is a short break, during which we review the information the parents have given, along with the child assessment findings to identify the factors that contribute to the onset of the stammer, its development and whether the child is vulnerable to persistent stammering. These factors are recorded on the case history form (see Appendix VIII) under the headings: 'physiological', 'speech and language', 'environmental' and 'psychological'.

Case study *Scott, aged three years*

Moderate stammer featuring whole- and part-word repetitions, prolongations and blocking.

Physiological factors

- *Family history of persistence*
- *Rapid speaking rate.*

Speech and language factors

- *Advanced receptive and expressive language skills.*

Environmental factors

- *Competition to speak with sister*
- *Parents' concern regarding openness about the stammering.*

Psychological factors

- *Scott sets himself high standards*
- *His sensitivity*
- *His tendency to worry and not talk about it*
- *His reaction to his stammering (giving up, looking away, 'I can't say it').*

There were no birth or developmental problems.

Case study *Khaled, aged five years*

Mild stammering featuring whole- and part-word repetitions and one prolongation.

Physiological factors

- *Family history of recovery*
- *Oro-motor skills*
- *Tiredness*
- *Rapid speaking rate.*

Speech and language factors

- *Speech sound difficulty*
- *Mismatch between speech and language skills*
- *Managing two languages.*

Environmental factors

- *Behaviour management.*

Psychological factors

- *Reduced confidence.*

The Summary Chart

The relevant information is then transferred to the top section of the Summary Chart (see Appendix III), so that, together with the information from the child assessment, it gives a representation of all the relevant issues in the child's breakdown of fluency.

The middle section of the Summary Chart (see Figure 4.3), which gives general aims of what the child needs, is then reviewed in light of the case history to ensure that the aims are appropriate.

Case study *Scott, aged three years*

Scott's needs:

1. *To take the pressure off himself by giving himself more time, using shorter, simpler utterances and not setting himself standards which are too high.*
2. *To be able to express his feelings.*
3. *To have a system of turn-taking with his sister.*

Case study *Khaled, aged five years*

Khaled's needs:

1 To give himself more time.

2 To have enough sleep to ensure that he is not tired.

3 To develop his phonological skills.

The bottom section of the Summary Chart (see Figure 4.6) is then completed to indicate which specific strategies will be targeted in therapy.

Interaction strategies

Following the child assessment the PCI video was analysed to identify which interaction strategies would be helpful for the child's fluency, whether there was evidence of the parents already using these strategies and which strategies the parents might need to develop further. The case history may have highlighted other useful interaction strategies. For example, if the parents described the child as lacking in confidence and tending to let others sort things out for him, a helpful interaction strategy might be to follow the child's lead, letting him solve any problems and using praise and encouragement (see Figure 4.6).

Family strategies

These strategies are selected according to the specific factors identified and indicated in the top section of the Summary Chart. For example, if the parents reported that the child stammers less when he is well-rested, but they are finding it difficult to settle him to bed at night, the 'Sleep' section is ticked in the 'Family strategies' column.

Child strategies

These strategies are introduced after the indirect component (interaction and family strategies) of Palin PCI. They are also selected according to the specific factors identified and indicated in the top section of the Summary Chart. For example, the child may present with delayed phonological development and therefore needs direct therapy to focus on developing his speech sounds.

When we have completed the Summary Chart, it gives us a representation of the factors which may be contributing to the child's stammer, as well as an individualised therapy plan for the child and family. We feed back this information to the parents in the formulation, as described in Chapter 5.

See Appendices IX and X for completed Summary Charts for Scott and Khaled.

(a)

Interaction strategies	Helpful	Evidence of Mother	Evidence of Father	Potential target Mother	Potential target Father
Following child's lead in play	✓	✓	✓	✓	
Letting child solve problems					
More comments than questions	✓	✓	✓		
Complexity of questions at child's level	✓	✓	✓		
Language is appropriate to child's level	✓	✓	✓		
Language is semantically contingent on child's focus	✓	✓	✓		
Repetition, expansion, rephrasing					
Time to initiate, respond, finish	✓	✓	✓	✓	✓
Rate of input when compared with child's rate	✓	✓	✓		✓
Use of pausing	✓	✓	✓	✓	✓
Using eye contact, position, touch, humour and/or surprise	✓	✓	✓	✓	
Praise and encouragement	✓	✓	✓		

Family strategies	
Special Times	✓
Managing two languages	
Openness about stammering	✓
Building confidence	✓
Turn-taking	✓
Dealing with feelings	✓
High standards	✓
Sleep	
Behaviour management	
Routines	
Pace of life	
Emerging issues	

Child strategies	
Rate reduction	✓
Pausing to think	✓
Easy onset	
Being more concise	
Eye contact/ focus of attention	
Other	
Language/phonology therapy	
School/preschool liaison	
Onward referral	

(b)

Interaction strategies	Helpful	Evidence of Mother	Evidence of Father	Potential target Mother	Potential target Father
Following child's lead in play	✓	✓		✓	
Letting child solve problems	✓				
More comments than questions	✓	✓			
Complexity of questions at child's level	✓	✓			
Language is appropriate to child's level	✓	✓			
Language is semantically contingent on child's focus	✓	✓			
Repetition, expansion, rephrasing	✓	✓		✓	
Time to initiate, respond, finish	✓	✓		✓	
Rate of input when compared with child's rate	✓	✓		✓	
Use of pausing	✓	✓		✓	
Using eye contact, position, touch, humour and/or surprise	✓	✓			
Praise and encouragement	✓	✓			

Family strategies	
Special Times	✓
Managing two languages	✓
Openness about stammering	
Building confidence	✓
Turn-taking	
Dealing with feelings	
High standards	
Sleep	✓
Behaviour management	✓
Routines	
Pace of life	
Emerging issues	

Child strategies	
Rate reduction	✓
Pausing to think	✓
Easy onset	
Being more concise	
Eye contact/ focus of attention	
Other	
Language/phonology therapy	✓
School/preschool liaison	
Onward referral	

FIGURE 4.6 Interaction, family and child strategies for (a) Scott (aged three) and (b) Khaled (aged five)

Troubleshooting

My manager is concerned about the amount of time spent on the assessment

Although we acknowledge that the full assessment may involve more time than typically allocated to a routine initial assessment, we know from clinical experience that the extra time invested at the initial stages is both efficient and cost-effective. We are more likely to fully understand the factors which are contributing to the child's stammer and provide the most appropriate intervention.

I am worried that parents may not want to be videoed

Therapists sometimes express concern about how parents may react to being video-recorded. Although occasionally a parent may say that they are feeling a little anxious about being video-recorded, in our experience this rarely happens. We have found that when a therapist explains to a parent in a matter of fact way what is going to happen, and how the video will help, parents have no difficulties with the task. We have worked with many families from different cultural groups and have used the video during both assessment and therapy as recommended.

I don't think that both parents will be able to attend

For many years we have advocated the inclusion of both parents (where appropriate) or main carers in the assessment and management of the child who stammers. Our position is that we are more effective if we involve both parents in the assessment and therapy process. We have found that when both parents understand the issues, they can work together to make the child's home environment conducive to fluency. We would therefore always recommend that both parents are *required* to participate in the process.

As indicated earlier, there are circumstances where this is inappropriate and we make alternative arrangements in such situations.

In our experience, if parents understand the reasons why they are both required to attend with the child, most will make the necessary arrangements. If they cannot, assessment and therapy can proceed but it may have less effect and take longer. Therapists report that they have been more successful in encouraging both parents to attend when they feel more confident about the rationale and are able to explain the reasons to parents. Therapists have also reported an increase in both parents attending when appointment letters state that both parents are *required* to attend rather than both parents are *encouraged* to attend.

However, we acknowledge the difference between running a busy, generalist clinic and a specialist centre. At a specialist centre, most parents are anxious to do whatever is required, especially if they have had a struggle or a wait for an appointment. During our teaching of speech & language therapists in the UK, we brainstorm why it is important to include both parents and a long list of ideas is typically generated.

No video camera

If no video camera is available, the evaluation may be done 'live', but this can be difficult as there is no opportunity to check out observations by reviewing the material. Another alternative to a video recording is an audio recording, but this gives no visual information about non-verbal aspects of the evaluation.

A video camera is an invaluable tool for an SLT in the assessment and management of a wide range of speech and language disorders. Making video recordings of our own clinical practice is also very useful in reflective practice and supervision. If the SLT does not have a video, we recommend that a request is made to purchase one, and good quality cameras are available for a reasonable cost. If equipment cannot be purchased, it is possible that the SLT service may have one available for loan, or some clinics have systems available for their staff. Alternatively, it is possible that the family you are working with have their own camera, which could be used in the sessions.

5

Formulation

The full assessment will have generated information about factors that contribute to the onset of the stammer, its development and whether the child is vulnerable to persistent stammering. The Summary Chart (Appendix III) gives a representation of all these factors, together with the possible range of strategies which will inform the treatment plan.

The 'formulation' is the way in which we assimilate the relevant information in order to give parents a clear and logical explanation of the child's stammering. It is based on the multifactorial model and offers the rationale for our recommendations.

We know that parents are more likely to engage fully in the therapy process when they understand more about stammering and how they can help their child. This understanding will often reduce the parents' levels of anxiety about the stammering.

How to make the formulation accessible

Developing the formulation in a way that is accessible, positive and memorable for any parent is clearly important. The following strategies may be helpful.

Use plain English

Jargon is useful and efficient between professionals, but if others do not understand it, it is of little value. The use of plain English is our aim and our responsibility.

Use parents' words

We use the parents' own words when referring back to the case history information as this will validate their comments and insights. Using their terms of reference will also ensure clear communication, for example:

'You said...

- *"It's like his brain is going too fast for his mouth."*
- *"His mouth is in action before his brain is in gear."*
- *"He's really sensitive – he feels things more than his brother."*
- *"She's a real perfectionist and always has to have things just right."'*

Include positive information to get the balance right

There is a danger that the formulation might become a depressing catalogue of the child's and family's difficulties and challenges. We make a point of feeding back genuine, positive aspects about the child and the family, affirming the parents whenever possible, for example:

- 'It is clear that you are very caring parents.'
- 'You have been through some very tough times but you are determined to do the best you can for your child.'
- 'You've already been very proactive about seeking help and are making good use of the help you've been offered.'
- 'He was so friendly and funny, he settled really quickly and then concentrated for a really long time.'

Check that you are making sense

It is usually possible to tell, just by looking at the parents, if they understand or agree with what we are saying during the formulation. Their body language indicates whether we are making sense or if they are puzzled. We check with them at regular intervals, for example *'Am I getting this right?', 'Is this making any sense?', 'Do you want me to clarify that?'*

Encourage the parents to ask you questions

We encourage parents to tell us if we say something that they do not understand or do not agree with. It is also helpful if they feel able to ask questions to help them clarify their understanding of any aspect of the formulation. However, if they are getting side-tracked, we suggest that we will return to this question after the feedback about their child.

A parents' handout for use during the formulation may be found in Appendix XI.

Handout for parents:
General facts about stammering

Format of the formulation

General facts about stammering

We begin with some general information, as listed on the parents' handout:

- Stammering has been around for centuries and, throughout history, many famous people stammered, such as King George VI, Marilyn Monroe, Winston Churchill and, more recently, Rowan Atkinson, Bruce Willis and Tiger Woods.
- It occurs across the world and it is more common in boys than girls.
- Stammering tends to start between the ages of two and four, at a time when speech and language are developing.
- Research has shown that about five per cent of children start to stammer and one per cent continue to stammer into adult life. That means that approximately four out of five children will overcome the difficulty. Research is helping us work out which children are most likely to persist and what sorts of therapy may help.
- Stammering is a complicated problem because there is no single cause of stammering and no simple cure.

Feedback from child assessment

We summarise the findings from the child assessment for the parents, starting with positive comments, for example about his social skills, co-operation or concentration. We describe the stammering behaviours noticed in the assessment, the amount of stammering and the child's insight, awareness and his level of concern. We also feed back the results of the speech and language tests, together with any informal observations. As described above, we link this to any comments or observations that the parents have made during the case history. We then apply these child assessment findings to the multifactorial model, as described below.

Why some children stammer

We briefly explain the research into possible factors which influence the onset and development of stammering, showing the parents the multifactorial model (see Figure 1.1) on their handout (see Appendix XI).

How much we say will depend on our judgement about what is important to a particular family and how much time is available. It is important that parents understand stammering in relation to their child.

An example of the wording of a formulation

General points:

- We know that stammering is likely to be the result of a combination of factors. This is why we call it 'multifactorial'. These factors vary between children.
- We have divided them into physiological, speech and language, environmental and psychological factors. Some factors explain why a child starts to stammer and others may help us to understand why he continues.

Physiological factors

Genetics

Research has shown that about two out of three people who stammer have a history of stammering in the family. This research also shows that if the relative has stopped stammering by the time he is an adult, the child is more likely to overcome the stammering:

'In your child's case the fact that he has an uncle who stammered as a child shows us that he was born with a tendency to stammer but he has also inherited the likelihood of getting better.'

'There is a family history of stammering into adulthood - you said that your uncle and your father both stammer, and you feel that you still stammer when you are under pressure. So your child may have inherited this tendency. This doesn't mean he will definitely keep stammering, because we know that helping him at this stage can be very effective.'

Speech motor skills

Some research studies have shown differences in the speech motor skills of some people who stammer – these may be slightly slower or less well co-ordinated and therefore they need to give themselves more time to plan and produce speech:

'You said that your child can be a messy eater and his speech is not very clear, so it is possible that his oral skills are still developing, and this may be one factor which is affecting his fluency.'

'Your child doesn't seem to have any trouble with his oral skills - he eats and chews well and his speech has always been very clear.'

Brain functioning research

Most researchers now consider stammering to have an underlying neurological cause that interferes with the production of speech and language. Studies in adults who stammer suggest that there may be some differences in the structure of their brains, as well as how they process speech and language. However, it is not yet clear if these differences have happened as a result of the stammering. These experiments cannot be used with young children so at the moment we cannot tell if the differences might cause the stammering, but one day perhaps this research may help us to understand more about why children start to stammer:

'There is also a lot of research into the brain structure and function of adults who stammer. They have found some differences between the brains of people who stammer and those who don't, but what we don't yet know is whether these differences are the result of years of stammering or the initial cause. Only when these studies are done with very young children who stammer will we know whether these differences cause stammering. So it is possible that the wiring of your child's brain may be different, which is making it harder for him to be fluent.'

Speech and language factors

Many children who stammer have normally developing speech and language skills, others have delayed language development and some are advanced.

Sometimes, different aspects of a child's linguistic ability are developing at a different pace. Research has shown that these mismatches in speech and language skills may be contributing to the stammering.

We also know from research that for some children the longer and more complicated their sentences are, the more likely they are to stammer:

'The assessments showed that your child's understanding of language is very well developed and he has a very wide spoken vocabulary, but we also know his speech sounds are still developing. You also said that you feel he goes too fast for himself. All of these facts may be contributing to the stammering.'

'You said that your child started to speak very late, and yet in the language assessments we did he was a bit ahead of his age. It seems that he has been through a period of very rapid language development, and this might have put some pressure on his fluency.'

'In the assessment we noticed that he sometimes finds it hard to think of the word he is trying to say. This might be causing his fluency to break down, especially when he is trying to say something in a hurry.'

Environmental factors

The home and school environments are important to consider in terms of how they might be affecting the child's stammer:

'Your child has a loving and stable home environment which is really supporting his fluency. You have a big family and what you have described as a very busy life. You said that he stammers more when he is competing with his sisters to talk and when he is in a rush. These things may be putting his fluency under pressure and we will discuss what we can do to help as a part of the therapy.'

'You have all been through some upheaval with the separation and then sorting out the custody arrangements. It has been hard for you all and you noticed that his stammering has been worse throughout all this. Children's fluency can be affected by strains and stresses and we will see what we can do to help settle things down in our therapy sessions.'

'We sometimes find that when a child is learning more than one language, his fluency can be affected. This doesn't mean that learning two languages has caused him to stammer in the first place; there will be other reasons for that. But managing both languages may just be making it a bit harder for him to speak fluently so we may look at how we can help your child to cope with this a bit better.'

'Your child has found settling into preschool quite difficult. This could be because he is used to it just being the two of you, and he's taking some time to adjust. The fact that he is feeling unsettled and a bit anxious may be affecting his fluency at the moment.'

Psychological factors

Each child who stammers is different in terms of his personality and some research has shown that children who stammer may be more sensitive. A child's personality will influence how he copes with a stammer:

'You described your child as being happy and carefree. He doesn't seem to be one of the sensitive ones, which is helpful, as he is likely to be less aware of his stammering or any reactions to it.'

'You said that he is a real worrier and he hates anyone being cross or upset. He sounds like quite a sensitive child, which may be affecting his speech at times.'

'You said that he is really aware of his stammering and he sometimes gives up on what he was going to say. You also said that he likes to have things just so and he hates getting things wrong. So it is possible that he is aware that he is not getting his speech quite right and this anxiety about it might be making it worse.'

Summary

'So, you can see that there are a number of issues that may be making your child vulnerable: the family history; the mismatch between his sophisticated language skills and his developing speech skills; his tendency to go a bit too fast for himself; the competition to speak and the busy family life. However, we know that his uncle grew out of the problem; your child has a lovely family life; and he is not particularly sensitive about his speech or anything else.

Therapy sessions are aimed at reducing some of those vulnerabilities so that we can build up his fluency and increase his chances of overcoming the stammering.'

Recommendations and management

The formulation should underpin the rationale for therapy – some of the factors that seem to be relevant for understanding the child's stammering also indicate areas for intervention. It is helpful if therapy can be arranged to start soon after the formulation, while the parents have a clear understanding of the relevant issues and the therapeutic relationship is established.

Each child will have an individually tailored therapy package, which will typically consist of interaction and family strategies, with subsequent child or other strategies as necessary.

The therapy is described in general terms so that parents will understand their role and the commitment involved:

'I would like to arrange a course of Palin Parent-Child Interaction therapy for you both with your child. I will need the three of you to come once a week for six weeks. Each session will last one hour.

In the sessions we will be looking at what helps your child to be fluent, and working out how we can build on this. We will use the video to help us find ways in which you can interact with him that will help his fluency. It is important for the therapy to be carried on at home, so I will ask you to practise these things at home each week. We will also discuss other ways in which the family can help his fluency.

At the end of the six weeks we start the home consolidation period. During this time you will carry on all the things you have been doing and we will keep in touch about how it is going.

At the end of this consolidation phase, you will come back with your child and we will discuss whether he has made sufficient progress, or if we need to do some more therapy.'

Clinical report

At the MPC we write an evidence-based report, outlining the relevant findings from the child assessment and case history, and describing the recommended treatment plan. This is sent to the parents in the first instance for them to check, clarify or request changes. Copies are then distributed to relevant people, as agreed with the parents. Local primary care trusts and other employers will have their own systems and policies relating to clinical reports.

Important questions that parents sometimes ask

- 'Will he grow out of it?'

We don't know for sure. Research is beginning to show us which children are more likely to continue to stammer and which might grow out of it, but these are only guidelines. We do know that early intervention is most effective so it is great that you have brought your child in at this stage so that we can give him the best chance. The good news is that he..., but we have to be realistic about his vulnerability to persistence.

- 'Is there a cure?'

Not at this stage. Nobody has found one way of treating stammering which works for everyone who stammers. You may hear of someone saying that he has been cured, but what worked for him may not suit others. That is why we do such a thorough assessment, to find out what each individual child will need to help him with his particular difficulties.

- 'Does this mean he has brain damage?'

No, we don't think children who stammer have brain damage, but in the future we may find out if there are some differences in the way in which their brains work. Maybe they are wired a bit differently, we do not know. But we do know ways of helping them to become more fluent, no matter what is going on in their brains.

- 'Why does stammering vary so much?'

It is a great puzzle. One moment a child can say what he wants with no trouble at all and the next he is stammering, with no obvious explanation. Or he may have weeks of being fluent and then the stammer is back for no apparent reason. It is possible that it is linked with these spurts in learning and growing that we see in all children. The trouble is, often we don't realise there has been a spurt until after the event!

'How many therapy sessions will he need?'

In the first instance, we will book six sessions and then you will practise at home for six weeks. You will then come back in for a review session, when we can decide if he needs any more therapy. For many children, all we need to do at that stage is see them from time to time to keep an eye on things. If we decide he needs more therapy we will book more sessions in, but it will not be week-in, week-out for ever, we will do blocks of therapy and monitor his progress.

Case study *Scott, aged three years*

Scott's parents were each given a copy of the handout for parents.

General facts about stammering

The parents were referred to the relevant section on the handout.

Feedback from child assessment

Scott did really well during his assessment. He was very co-operative and he concentrated throughout all the different tasks we did. He was friendly and chatty and I enjoyed assessing him.

He scored really highly in all the language tests. He's only three and he came out at over a five-year level, so you were right in thinking that he has good language skills – they are excellent. I noticed he talked a lot and his sentences were often long and complicated. As you said, he does tend to talk quickly and it often comes out in a burst of fast talking.

He did stammer during the assessment and I saw the same kinds of stammering that you described – repetitions of sounds and words, prolongations (where he stretches out the sounds) and blocking (where nothing comes out). I did not see any of the extra movements you talked about, such as clenching his fists, but maybe that is because he was just in the one-to-one setting with me. I calculated the percentage of his stammering, which came out as 9.8 per cent, meaning that he stammered on nearly 10 in every 100 syllables. It also means he was 90 per cent fluent. We rate this amount and type of stammering as being moderate.

I asked him about how he was getting on with his talking and he said 'I can't say my words.' When I asked him some more questions he did not say much. Maybe his concentration had run out by then or he did not want to talk about his speech. Anyway, he is obviously aware of the stammering, just as you said. I also noticed some of that carefulness and tidiness you described, like putting the pictures in a perfectly straight line! Also, he was checking with me from time to time about how he was getting on, so, just as you said, he is keen to do well.

Why some children stammer

We know that stammering is likely to be the result of a combination of factors. This is why we call it 'multifactorial'. These factors vary between children, and this assessment has helped me to understand what Scott's factors might be. As you can see on this diagram [see Figure 1.1], we have divided them into physiological, speech and language, environmental and psychological. Some factors explain why a child starts to stammer and others may show why it continues.

First, the physiological factors.

- *Research has shown that about two out of three people who stammer have a history of stammering in the family. This research also shows that if the relative has stopped stammering by the time he is an adult, the child is more likely to overcome the stammering. In Scott's case he has quite a strong family history of stammering. You [father] stammered as a child and you say that you still do when you are under a bit of pressure. You also found out that your father and your uncle stammered into adulthood. This tells us that Scott may have inherited this tendency (although it is not a certainty, and his twin sister inherited the same tendency and doesn't stammer). It also means that he might continue to stammer.*
- *There is also a lot of research into the brain structure and function of adults who stammer. They have found some differences between the brains of people who stammer and those who don't, but what we do not yet know is whether these differences are the result of years of stammering or the initial cause. Only when these studies are done with very young children who stammer will we know whether these differences cause stammering. So it is possible that the wiring of Scott's brain may be different, which is making it harder for him to be fluent.*
- *Some research studies have shown differences in the speech motor skills of some people who stammer – these may be slightly slower or less well co-ordinated. Scott does not seem to have any trouble with his speech motor skills – he eats and chews well and his speech has always been very clear.*

Second, the speech and language factors.

- *There is an overlap between the physiological and the speech and language factors, and this is where we think about a child's speed of talking. We have all commented on Scott's fast speech and this may be another thing that is making it harder for him to speak fluently: he just is not giving himself enough time.*
- *Many children who stammer have normally developing speech and language skills, others have delayed language development and some are advanced. In Scott's case, he is clearly advanced, which is a great asset. He is functioning two years ahead of himself – he has got a five-year-old brain*

and a three-year-old mouth. But this is putting enormous pressure on his fluency. When he adds to that pressure by talking very fast then his system is even more likely to break down. We also know from research that, for some children, the longer and more complicated their sentences are, the more likely they are to stammer.

Third, the environmental factors.

- *The home and school environments are important to consider in terms of how they might be affecting the child's stammer. Scott has a loving and stable home environment, which is really supporting his fluency. You said that he stammers more when he is competing with his sister to talk and when he is in a rush. These things may be putting his fluency under pressure and we will discuss what we can do to help as a part of the therapy.*
- *You also mentioned that you were worried about whether you should talk to Scott about his stammering, and how to do that. You said that he is aware he is doing it and maybe he is showing signs of worrying about it. So maybe there is a general anxiety around when he is stammering that we need to help you all with.*

Lastly, the psychological factors.

- *Some research has shown that children who stammer may be more sensitive. You have said that Scott is one of the sensitive ones and also that he is quite a worrier, but he does not tell you what is bothering him. He is also quite competitive and he puts himself under a lot of pressure to do well and get things right. When it comes to his speech, maybe his sensitivity and his perfectionism mean that he is more likely to notice when it is not quite right and this really bothers him, but he is keeping all these feelings to himself. So maybe we can think of ways to manage all of that, which might reduce the stammering.*

To summarise, then, there is no one cause of Scott's stammering and you certainly did not cause it. He was born with a likelihood of stammering and his excellent language skills, together with his fast pace, have probably triggered the problem. When that is combined with competing with his sister to talk, and his emotions getting fired up, the stammering is more likely to happen.
Does that make any sense to you?
Was there anything that you didn't agree with?
Would you like to ask me about any of it?

Case study *Khaled, aged five years*

Khaled's mother was given a copy of the handout for parents.

General facts about stammering

She was referred to the relevant section on the handout.

Feedback from child assessment

Khaled did really well during his assessment. He seemed a bit shy at first, but he settled quickly and co-operated and concentrated well. He took turns well and used eye contact appropriately.

He did very well in all the language tests. Many children who are learning two languages are a bit behind in their language development, but his understanding and use of English is right for his age, just as you said in the case history. You also said that some of his speech sounds were wrong, and I noticed that, too. I could understand him once I was used to it, and the mistakes he is making are common in younger children. You are right that he talks fast, and it is harder to understand him when he does that.

Khaled did stammer during the assessment and I saw the same kinds of stammering that you described – repetitions of sound and words, prolongations (where he stretches out the sounds). I calculated the percentage of his stammering, which came out as six per cent, meaning that he stammered on six in every 100 syllables. We rate this amount and type of stammering as being mild.

When I asked Khaled about how he was getting on with his talking I think he had had enough, but even so I think you are right that he is not aware of any difficulty.

Why some children stammer

We know that stammering is likely to be the result of a combination of factors. This is why we call it 'multifactorial'. These factors vary between children, and this assessment has helped me to understand what Khaled's factors might be.

As you can see on this diagram [see Figure 1.1], we have divided them into physiological, speech and language, environmental and psychological. Some factors explain why a child starts to stammer and others may show why it continues.

First, the physiological factors.

- *Research has shown that about two out of three people who stammer have a history of stammering in the family. This research also shows that if the relative has stopped stammering by the time he is an adult, the child is more likely to overcome the stammering. In Khaled's case there is a family history of stammering. Your brother stammered as a child, but he grew out of it. Khaled may have inherited the tendency to stammer (although it is not a certainty, and his brother inherited the same tendency and he does not stammer). But it also means that he has inherited the tendency to grow out of it, which is encouraging.*

- *There is also a lot of research into the brain structure and function of adults who stammer. They have found some differences between the brains of people who stammer and those who do not, but what we do not yet know is whether these differences are the result of years of stammering or the initial cause. Only when these studies are done with very young children who stammer will we know whether these differences cause stammering. So it is possible that the wiring of Khaled's brain may be different, which is making it harder for him to be fluent.*
- *Some research studies have shown differences in the speech motor skills of some people who stammer – these may be slightly slower or less well co-ordinated. You described Khaled as a messy eater, and we know that his speech sounds are not quite right, so it seems possible that he is having some trouble with co-ordinating his mouth when he eats and speaks. This may be contributing to his stammering.*

Second, the speech and language factors.

- *There is an overlap between the physiological and the speech and language factors, and this is where we think about a child's speed of talking. We've both commented on Khaled's fast speech and this may be another thing that is making it harder for him to speak fluently: he just is not giving himself enough time.*
- *Many children who stammer have normally developing speech and language skills, others have delayed language development and some are advanced. Sometimes, different aspects of a child's linguistic ability are developing at a different pace. Research has shown that these mismatches in speech and language skills may be contributing to the stammering. In Khaled's case, his language skills are appropriate for his age, but his speech sounds are still developing, so there is a mismatch which may be affecting his fluency.*

Third, the environmental factors.

- *The home and school environments are important to consider in terms of how they might be affecting the child's stammer. Khaled has a loving and stable home environment, which is really supporting his fluency. It must be hard for you sometimes to manage on your own, but you have clearly done a great job in bringing up such a friendly and likeable child.*
- *You talked about the difficulties you sometimes have with his behaviour, especially at bedtime, and you are linking this to him stammering more. So it seems a good idea to think about how to manage these issues in our therapy, so that we can help his speech.*

Lastly, the psychological factors.

- *Some research has shown that children who stammer may be more sensitive than children who do not stammer. Khaled does not seem to be one of the sensitive ones, nor is he a worrier, which is great because these things can affect children's fluency. You did mention that he might be less confident at preschool so maybe we can help with that in our therapy.*

To summarise then, there is no one cause of Khaled's stammering and you certainly did not cause it. He was born with a likelihood of stammering, and his oral skills are still developing, so these things have probably triggered the problem. When that is combined with him talking fast, or getting tired or frustrated, the stammering is more likely to happen.
Does that make any sense to you?
Was there anything that you didn't agree with?
Would you like to ask me about any of it?

Interaction Strategies

6

Palin Parent–Child Interaction therapy

In this chapter we discuss our therapeutic style of working with parents and the importance of building an alliance with them. The format of the programme will then be presented on a session-by-session basis.

The Palin Parent–Child Interaction style

Palin PCI aims to enable parents to build on their knowledge and develop their skills in the use of interaction and family strategies to maximise their child's fluency. We want to do this in a way that will empower and equip parents, and reduce their anxieties.

Building on knowledge: asking, not telling

We have moved away from the traditional or medical 'expert' model of telling parents what to do. Instead we elicit their insights and their instinctive understanding, and develop their valuable knowledge and skills.

For example, instead of telling parents what we think seems to affect a child's fluency (time pressure, his emotional state or linguistic complexity), we ask parents about their observations:

- 'What seems to help your child to be more fluent?'
- 'When is his speech better?'
- 'When does he stammer more?'
- 'What do you think he needs to do to stammer less?'
- 'What do you do or say to help him when he is stammering?'
- 'How do you think that is helping him?'

We use these questions repeatedly throughout our therapy programme and we have found that, typically, parents can answer these questions because they know their child and what affects him. Drawing this knowledge from them is empowering and memorable.

Developing skills: discovering, not showing

When we model how to do something, parents might feel they could never do it as well as they should. When we identify examples of when parents are already using their skills to help their child's fluency, this increases their confidence in their own ability. For example, instead of showing a parent how to match their linguistic complexity to the child's level, by the therapist playing with the child and talking to him at the appropriate level, we look at a recording with the parent and ask them to find an instance of when they are using the appropriate level.

The Palin PCI format

Palin PCI is carried out in a block of six once-weekly sessions for one hour, followed by a six-week home consolidation period and then a review appointment. This format is compatible with most generalist clinic treatment schedules. We involve both parents, as appropriate, and the child.

The full assessment has equipped us with a profile of the child's abilities and vulnerabilities. The interaction analysis has identified:

- which interaction strategies might facilitate the child's fluency
- which interaction strategies the parents are already using and which they could build on.

In Palin PCI sessions, parents watch video recordings of themselves playing with their child. They learn to identify and discuss what they are already doing to support the child's fluency and then they practise developing these strategies. Home practice sessions are set up within the framework of brief, regular 'Special Times'.

Incorporated into the course of Palin PCI is a programme for developing the child's confidence, based on the Faber and Mazlish (1980) model. In addition to this, other family strategies identified in the full assessment are addressed as necessary. These could include turn-taking in the family, bedtime routines and behaviour management.

In order to carry out Palin PCI, the therapist will need:

- A room with play material suitable for the child's age and ability
- The first parent–child interaction videotape recording
- A video camera and connection leads
- A TV monitor
- Special Times instruction sheets (Session 1) (see Appendix XII)
- Special Times task sheets (all sessions) (see Appendix XIII)
- Parents' handouts, as appropriate (see Appendices XIV–XVIII).

Session 1:

- *Video recording if necessary*
- *Review assessment findings*
- *Describe therapy*
- *Set up Special Times*
- *If appropriate, discuss 'Managing two languages'*
- *If appropriate, give 'Openness about stammering' handout*

The therapy programme will now be described in a session-by-session format.

Session 1

Video recording of parent–child interaction, if required

If only one parent attended the child assessment, we make a video recording of the other parent during this first session. If there have been several months between assessment and therapy, we make a new video recording of both parents. Guidelines on setting up this recording can be found in Chapter 4.

Review of assessment findings

We revisit the outcome of the assessment with the parents, including the multifactorial framework and how it relates to their child. This provides the opportunity for clarification if the parents need it. It also helps to focus them on their child's profile of abilities and vulnerabilities, which will form the basis of Palin PCI. It is also an opportunity to follow up any other recommendations made during the formulation.

Description of therapy programme

We describe the format and aims of therapy in the following way

'As we discussed, we have arranged six once-weekly appointments which will last one hour. As we agreed, I will need [both of] you and your child to attend.

In the sessions we will do Palin Parent-Child Interaction therapy, which involves finding ways for you to help your child to become more fluent during play sessions. We will use video recordings to help us work out the best ways to help your child.

We will set up practice sessions to do at home, and task sheets to fill out.

We will also discuss other ways you can be helping your child at home in his daily life.

At the end of the six weeks, you will need to continue with the therapy at home for a further six weeks, without the weekly sessions here - this is called the consolidation period.

We do not expect to see an immediate improvement in your child's fluency. In fact, sometimes the child might stammer a bit more during the first six weeks of therapy. It is during the consolidation period that you usually see the benefits.

At the end of this time we will have a review appointment when we will discuss how your child is progressing and decide on what we should do next.'

Setting up Special Times

Special Times are central to Palin PCI. During Special Times parents focus on implementing their chosen interaction strategies, which we refer to as their 'targets', to help the child's fluency. They also provide an opportunity for 'quality time' for a child and parent to spend together. In this first session, we set up the Special Times. During the week that follows the parents will organise this within their family routine.

We explain to the parents that Special Times are central to the therapy process and we will spend this first session setting them up. The parents will then spend the first week making them part of their routine at home and, once this is established, we will incorporate strategies to help the child's fluency.

Handout:
Special Times instruction sheet

We give parents a copy of the 'Special Times instruction sheet' (see Appendix XII) to read and take home, and we explain the format of Special Times to the parents.

We then ask parents to make a commitment to do between three and five Special Times per week. Each parent has separate Special Times with the child and chooses how many he or she will do. They are then responsible for their own commitment. We encourage them to be realistic about how many Special Times they will be able to fit in. If they try to do too many they may find them difficult to implement. Conversely, we have found that fewer than three Special Times each per week is ineffective. A child may have more than one Special Time in a day, but not with the same parent. Some families prefer to have Special Times at regular times in the day, others adopt a more flexible approach. In a family with one parent and more than one child, we may need to be creative with the parent in thinking how to do the Special Times individually with their child.

Certain activities are not recommended, as these may not encourage verbal interaction, for example video games, reading or outdoor sports. We sometimes explore with parents the kinds of toys or games they have at home so that they feel confident about suitable activities for Special Times. It is the child who chooses the activity in Special Times, thus increasing his motivation to co-operate. If a mother has chosen her favourite puzzle there is a risk that the child will not want to play.

During Special Times, we encourage parents to focus on *what* the child is saying, not *how* he is saying it. We want parents to give their child their undivided attention and they should not be trying to do something else at the same time, such as cooking a meal or tidying the room. We may need to help the parents to decide where the Special Times should happen, a place where distractions or interruptions are unlikely.

We also suggest that parents do Special Times with their other children, to avoid the focus of attention being solely on the child who stammers.

Parents and children sometimes feel that five minutes is too brief, so we stress the importance of keeping to the time in the first week in order to establish the routine. Timers can be used to help a child who does not understand how long five minutes is. The five-minute limit is imposed for two reasons:

- It may be easier to find the opportunity for a Special Time if it is brief.
- It will be easier for a parent to focus on an aspect of their interaction style for five minutes. Any longer is difficult to maintain.

Handout:
'Special Times task sheet'

Once the parents have understood the Special Times task and have decided how many they will each do in a week, we give them a 'Special Times task sheet' (see Appendix XIII) to complete at home and bring back the following week. This provides a record of the Special Times and how the parents are getting on with practising their targets. We point out that the task sheets are not intended to be a record of the child's fluency. We write on the task sheet the number of Special Times each parent has agreed to do. We explain that in the first week the parents' target is to complete the agreed number of Special Times. In subsequent weeks, their targets will be different.

We explain to the parents that when they are ready to do the Special Times at home, they should ask the child if he is available for five minutes. They tell the child that after Special Times have finished they will have to write on their task sheet. After this they can then go back to playing with the child if they have time, but they let the child know that this is no longer Special Time.

Once the parents have understood the Special Times task, we explain it to the child, emphasising that he will choose the toy or activity, that it is only for five minutes and that the parents will have to write it down at the end:

'I have asked your mummy and daddy to do some homework for me. Do you think you could help them with their homework? They have to play with you for five minutes, which is actually a very short time. They will do this… times a week. We want you to choose what you want to play with (but not a book or the computer or television or doing sport). When the five minutes is finished, they have to write down what you did together on my sheet. So, do you think you could help them to do this?'

If the family strategy 'Managing two languages' has been identified as relevant during the assessment, we discuss this strategy with the parents in this first therapy session (see Chapter 7).

If the family strategy 'Openness about stammering' has been identified as relevant during the assessment, we give the parents this handout (see Chapter 7).

> ***Case study*** *Scott, aged three years*
>
> Session 1
>
> *As Scott's father had not been at the child assessment, we made a video recording of him playing with his son. We reviewed the assessment findings and the parents asked if it would be helpful for them to bring Scott's sister to the therapy sessions. It was suggested that she attend one session, when we would cover taking turns to speak.*
>
> *Before the Special Times instruction sheet was given, we asked Scott's mother whether her dyslexia would make it difficult to deal with written instructions, handouts or task sheets. She said that she would probably cope as long as it was not too complicated and she would ask if there was anything that she did not understand. She also said that her spelling was 'awful' but we reassured her that this did not matter. Scott's parents both chose to do three Special Times each with him and they were given the Special Times task sheets to complete and bring to the next session.*
>
> *Family strategy introduced: 'Openness about stammering' (see Chapter 7)*

> ***Case study*** *Khaled, aged five years*
>
> Session 1
>
> *We reviewed the assessment findings. Khaled's mother said she would do five Special Times with him. She was given a task sheet to complete and bring back to the next session.*
>
> *Family strategy introduced: 'Managing two languages' (see Chapter 7)*
>
> *Note: this session took around 20 minutes.*

Session 2

This session is critical in establishing the style of working with parents. The questions used here will be repeated in future sessions as they guide parents and tune them into what is needed to help the child.

Review of Special Times

> *Don't start PCI until Special Times are in place!*

At the beginning of each session we ask the parents to tell us about their Special Times and we read and keep the task sheets. If parents have completed their Special Times, therapy proceeds as below. However, if problems have arisen at this stage, they are discussed and Special Times are set up again,

Session 2:
- *Review Special Times*
- *Discuss child's abilities and what helps*
- *Watch video*
- *Make another video, if appropriate*
- *Set Special Times target*
- *Give task sheet*
- *If appropriate, discuss 'Openness about stammering'*

Before we watch the video:
- *What do we know about your child?*
- *What does he need to do to be more fluent?*
- *What are you already doing?*

without any targets being introduced. See the 'Troubleshooting' section at the end of this chapter.

Discuss the child's abilities and vulnerabilities and what might help

In order to elicit the parents' perceptions, we ask a series of questions (see 'Questions for the SLT to ask in Palin PCI sessions', Appendix XIX).

- Question 1: What have we found out about why your child stammers?

Before we watch the video, we focus on the child's abilities and vulnerabilities which affect his fluency. We ask parents to review what they already know about their child, as well as what we learnt from the assessment which may affect his fluency. For example, *Parents*: 'We know that he has good language skills, but his speech sound system is not right yet and he tends to talk quickly, especially when he is excited or in a group of people.'

- Question 2: What do you think he needs to do to be more fluent?

Having discussed the child's abilities and vulnerabilities, we then ask parents what they think helps the child to be more fluent. Parents may not realise that they already have this expertise about what helps their child; they are expecting us to give them this information. But they often have instincts about what might help: they might have wanted to tell the child to slow down, think about what he wants to say, calm down. These strategies are probably exactly what the child needs to do in order to be more fluent, but it might be difficult for the child to put this into practice. Palin PCI is designed to enable the parent to help the child do what he needs to do. For example, *Parents*: 'He needs to talk more slowly, give himself more time to get his tongue around what he is trying to say.'

- Question 3: What do you think you might already be doing that could be helping your child?

This question helps the parents to tap once again into their own expertise and knowledge, thinking about ways that they have *instinctively* been helping their child to do whatever helps him to be more fluent. For example:

'I let him finish what he is saying.'
'I try to keep calm so that he doesn't get flustered.'
'I tell him to take his time.'

Watch the parent–child interaction video

Before we watch the video with the parents, we say to the child that he can watch the video too, or he can play on his own for a while. We tell the parents that when they have watched the video, we will ask them how typical it is of them playing with their child and what they were doing to help their child's fluency. First, we play one parent's video clip and discuss it and then we do the same with the other parent's clip. Parents do not comment on each other's videos.

- Question 4: How typical is the video?

> **After we watch the video:**
> - *Is it typical?*
> - *What are you doing that helps his fluency?*
> - *How might that be helping?*
> - *What could you be doing more of?*

When they have watched the video, we ask each parent to comment on how typical his or her video is. This gives them the opportunity to tell us if they were uncomfortable about making the video or how they felt it went. We usually find that parents say the video is fairly typical. If parents say that the video is not really representative, we ask them to tell us about how it is different from what usually happens.

- Question 5: What are you doing that is helping your child's fluency?

We remind parents what they have told us is helpful for their child, for example:

'I let him finish what he is saying'
'I try to keep calm so that he doesn't get flustered'
'I tell him to take his time'

We then ask each parent if they noticed when they were using those helpful strategies on the video:

- Did you notice times when you were letting him finish? How did you do that?
- Were you sometimes helping him to keep calm?
- Did you notice times when you were helping him to take his time?

The video recording will provide useful examples of a parent using a helpful strategy, something we have already noted during the analysis of the PCI video. If the parents are finding it difficult to pick out examples of things that are going well, we replay these clips on the video.

Parents often find it uncomfortable to talk about what they are doing well, and are often quick to make negative observations. We redirect them to the positive aspects of their interaction. We can use the negative observation and turn it around.

For example:

Parent:	*'I am asking too many questions.'*
Therapist:	*'We all ask questions sometimes, especially when we are trying to get a child to talk. Did you notice when you said something that was not a question? [we show the parent a clip if necessary] What did you do instead of asking him something?'*

- Question 6: How might that be helping?

We then ask each parent how that particular strategy might be helping the child's fluency. For example: 'You noticed that you were helping him to take his time by speaking in a very laid-back way. How would this help his fluency?'

It is important that therapists know the rationale for working on an interaction strategy and why it helps a child's fluency. Information from research and clinical experience may be found at the end of this chapter.

- Question 7: What could you do more of?

From this discussion we agree with each parent one strategy that they will try to use as their target. Each parent decides on their own target. We may discuss in some detail ways that the parent can do this, as well as how it might help the child's fluency. Parent handouts are provided for the following strategies and may be a useful guide for this discussion:

- 'Letting my child take the lead in play' handout Appendix XIV
- 'Keeping things simple' handout Appendix XV
- 'Balancing comments and questions' handout Appendix XVI
- 'My rate of talking and use of pauses' handout Appendix XVII
- 'Eye contact and talking' handout Appendix XVIII.

We give these to the parents for them to further reflect at home on how that target might help the child's fluency and how they can implement it in their Special Times.

Make another video recording

We may ask the parents to do a brief practice of their target in the clinic. We record them playing for two to three minutes and then watch it. This gives them immediate feedback about their ability to develop their use of the target.

Set the Special Times target

We ask each parent to practise their chosen target in their Special Times with the child at home. We emphasise that, at this stage, parents are only expected to use their target during the Special Times, as it would be very difficult to focus on the target throughout their daily life.

Give the task sheets to parents

Each parent has their target written on their task sheet, as well as the number of Special Times they have agreed to do during the coming week. We ask them to write down on the sheet what they did in each Special Time, and add any comments they might have about using their target.

Discuss 'Openness about stammering'

See Chapter 7.

Case study *Scott, aged three years*

Session 2

Scott's parents had both completed their three Special Times and written brief notes on their task sheets. When asked about what we had found out in the assessment about Scott and his stammering, they recalled that his language skills were 'good for his age' and that he tended to speak very fast. They also said that he was worse when there was competition to speak, for example with his twin sister. They felt that in order to be more fluent he needed to take his time and 'keep it short and sweet.' They also thought that he needed to 'digest in his head' before he said something. Scott's mother said that she was already helping him by being 'at ease' herself, thereby putting him at ease. His father thought that he was already helping him by not rushing, because 'if you are in a rush, he rushes.' When they watched the video they both said they had felt self-conscious at the time, but, nevertheless, the video was a fairly typical picture of what they were like when they played with Scott. On the video, his mother noticed that she was giving him time to come up with what he wanted to say, rather than getting him to talk. She also thought that when she was looking at him he was 'at ease' because he knew he had her attention. She felt that this was helping his fluency because he was keeping calm and not rushing to speak. She agreed that in the Special Times at home she would focus on watching and waiting for Scott.

Scott's father initially said that he thought that his own speech sounded a bit rushed, because he was 'gabbling.' When the therapist replayed a number of clips on the video, he acknowledged that some of his speech was not rushed, it was 'slow and spaced out.' He decided that in his Special Times he would focus on keeping his speech slower and spaced out. Scott's mother was given the handout 'Letting my child take the lead in play' and his father was given 'My rate of talking and use of pauses.'

Family strategy discussed: 'Openness about stammering' (see Chapter 7)

Case study *Khaled, aged 5 years*

Session 2

Khaled's mother had done three Special Times and recorded these on the task sheet. She said that she had been able to do one after school each day while her older son was watching the television, but she had been ill for two days and at the weekend she found it very difficult to find the time to do a Special Time. She decided that she would aim to do three Special Times rather than five each week and any extras would be a bonus. For one of her Special Times she had written 'reading a book.' When she was asked to describe this, she said that Khaled had wanted to look at a book with her and they talked about the pictures. She was told that this was a good activity for a Special Time, because it meant that they could have a conversation, unlike just reading to Khaled, which she could do at other times.

When she was asked to reflect on what was contributing to Khaled's stammering, his mother said that it had been partly inherited from his uncle and also that his 'speech muscles' were not working properly. This was further discussed to clarify that he found it slightly difficult to co-ordinate all the rapid processes involved in talking. His mother said that it was 'like his brain is ahead of his mouth.' The therapist asked when this was particularly noticeable and she said when he was 'butting in' or arguing to get his own way. When she was asked what she felt Khaled needed to do to be more fluent, his mother said, 'take his time and not rush,' and she tried to help him to do this by saying 'slow down.' The video recording from the assessment was played and Khaled's mother said that she thought it was fairly typical of how they normally are together. When she was asked, ' What did you notice that you were doing on the video to help Khaled to slow down?,' she said that she hadn't noticed anything like that, but she was worried that her own speech sounded really fast. The video was replayed and clips were shown when she was matching Khaled's rate. When she was asked to describe what she was doing, Khaled's mother said she was talking more slowly. Her speech rate was compared with Khaled's and she said that she was actually a bit slower than him. She also noticed that she was good at waiting, 'giving him time to come up with his answer,' and that she was happy to allow silences, when neither of them said anything. There was a discussion about how these ideas were helpful for Khaled's fluency, and she decided that for her Special Times target she would make sure her talking was a bit slower than Khaled's. This target was written on her task sheet and she was given the handout 'My rate of talking and use of pauses.'

Family strategy discussed: 'Managing two languages' (see Chapter 7)

Sessions 3, 4 and 5

Sessions 3–5 of Palin PCI therapy follow the same format:

- Review of Special Times and task sheets
- Record the interaction video
- Watch the video and review the target or identify an additional target
- Set Special Times targets and give task sheets
- Make another video recording
- Discuss the family strategy
- Give the appropriate handout to introduce the next family strategy.

Review of Special Times and task sheets

We ask specifically about the Special Times, in particular how the parents managed with their target. We read through and retain the task sheets. Appendix XX gives an example of a completed task sheet.

Record the interaction video

We then ask each parent and the child to do a short Special Time in the clinic, showing their targeted change. We video record this for two or three minutes in order to provide the parents with feedback on their progress.

Watch the video and review the target or introduce an additional target

We watch the video recording with the parents and ask each of them to comment on their use of their target. Sometimes parents can be very negative in their observations, and we need to help them to focus on instances when they have used their target successfully.

It is usual for a parent to retain the same target for a number of weeks. However, sometimes they find it relatively easy to make more use of a target, and they report that they have started to use it throughout the day, not just in Special Times. We then help the parent to identify an additional target for change, using the same process as above, but making sure that the parents are not moving on too quickly to a new target. We would typically have a maximum of three targets during the first six sessions.

Set the Special Times targets and give task sheets

Each parent agrees their target(s) for Special Times, which are written on their task sheets for that week. If there is more than one target, all the targets are recorded on the sheet.

Make another video recording

If necessary, we ask the parents to do a brief practice of their target in the clinic, which we record and review with them.

Discuss the family strategy

Any family strategies are discussed, as appropriate (see Chapter 7).

Give the appropriate handout for the family strategy discussion for the following week

Handout:
Building my child's confidence

In Session 3 we would normally give the handout 'Building my child's confidence' (see Appendix XXI) in preparation for the next session when we will discuss the issue. Details of this are given in Chapter 7.

Case study *Scott, aged three years*

Session 3

Scott's mother reported that she had done three Special Times and she had written that she found it relaxing to use her target of watching and waiting for Scott. She noticed that he seemed very calm and they both enjoyed the Special Times. Scott's father had done just one Special Time as he had worked several night shifts and found it hard to find the time. Since this shift pattern was likely to happen again, we discussed ways that he might be able to fit in Special Times in a week when he was working nights. He agreed he would do one Special Time with Scott before going to work one evening, and the other two on his days off between shifts. Scott's father felt that the one Special Time he had done had gone well – he had found that he needed to concentrate hard on pausing and going a bit slower, but Scott hadn't noticed anything strange and they still had fun. A video recording was made of each parent using their target as they played with Scott. When she watched her video, his mother said that she was pleased with how she was just sitting back and letting Scott 'do his own thing'. She also noticed that she was allowing long silences, and when Scott did say something he seemed to have 'sorted it out in his head first'. She noticed that sometimes when she asked him questions or made a comment about what he was doing, she did not give him a chance to respond before she said something else. When she was shown clips of times when she did give him time to respond, she realised that she was already doing this and she wanted to do more of it. Her targets were set as 'watching and waiting' and 'giving Scott time to respond before I say something else'. She was given a copy of the handout 'My rate of talking and use of pauses'. Scott's dad noticed that he was going much slower on his video. He said that he wanted to keep this as his target as it did not come naturally and he wanted to practise it a lot more. As usual, they were given Special Times task sheets with their targets written on them.

Family strategy reviewed: 'Openness about stammering'

Family strategy introduced: 'Building my child's confidence'

Session 4

Both parents had completed their Special Times and Scott's father commented that he had found that he was consciously talking more slowly at other times too. A video recording was made of each of them playing with Scott and we watched the tape. His mother was pleased that she was giving Scott lots of time to say something or to respond when she said something and she commented that he was much more fluent during his Special Times. She had also noticed this on the clinic video recording. She decided to keep her current targets. Scott's father said that his own speech sounded much slower in his head than it did on the video. There was a clip on the video when Scott asked him a question and he paused for a couple of seconds before answering. This was shown to Scott's father and he was asked what was particularly helpful about it. He commented that he actually was taking a moment to think, and he realised that this was a good thing to do with Scott, as he might follow his father's example. He decided that his targets would be 'going more slowly' and 'waiting for a moment before speaking'. Both parents were given Tasks Sheets with their targets recorded.

Family strategy discussed: 'Building my child's confidence'

Family strategy introduced: 'Turn-taking'

Session 5

Scott attended Session 5 with his twin sister and his parents. His mother said that they had had a difficult week because both the children and she had had flu, so she hadn't done any Special Times. Scott's father had done one. They had noticed that Scott had started to stammer more when he was ill but they felt that his speech was a bit better now. It was agreed that now everyone was well again they would reinstate the Special Times, three times a week and maintaining their current targets. They were given Tasks Sheets.

Family strategy reviewed: 'Building my child's confidence'

Family strategy discussed: 'Turn-taking'

Family strategy introduced: 'Dealing with feelings' and 'The child whose standards are too high'

Case study *Khaled, aged five years*

Session 3

Khaled's mother had done four Special Times and completed the task sheets. She said that she found it quite easy to talk a bit slower than Khaled in the Special Times, but she could not remember to do it for the rest of the time. She was reassured that she was not expected to do it at any time except during Special Times at this early stage. A video recording was made and it was noticed that she was talking more slowly, and she commented that Khaled seemed to be 'a bit calmer and steadier'. She decided to continue with this target for another week and was given the task sheet.

Family strategy introduced: 'Building my child's confidence'

Session 4

At Session 4, Khaled's mother reported that she had done five Special Times. A video recording was made of them playing 'Pop up Pirate', when they both became quite excited. When she watched the video Khaled's mother noticed that she was still using a slower rate, even though she was excited. She thought that sometimes they almost 'talked over' each other when the tension was building. Clips of the video were shown when she was pausing between Khaled speaking and her reply. She decided that she would have an additional target of trying to do this more.

Family strategy discussed: 'Building my child's confidence'

Family strategy introduced: 'Bedtimes'

Session 5

Khaled's mother said she had only been able to do three Special Times as both the boys had been ill and life was all out of routine, but she had made a special effort to try out her targets at other times when she was talking to Khaled. She had noticed that he was stammering a bit more, possibly because he was ill, and so she tried to use the pausing and slower rate when she spoke to him. She was praised for doing this, especially because the normal routines were not in place. A video recording was made and she noticed that she was often repeating what Khaled was saying before she responded to it. This was discussed in relation to how it might be helping his speech sound development. Khaled's mother decided that she was giving him a clear model of how he should pronounce a word. It was pointed out that this was particularly helpful because she was not correcting him, or asking him to repeat it after her. She would not be putting his fluency under pressure by making him focus too much on how to say sounds, but he would hear a correct version of the word. Khaled's mother decided that she would try to do more repeating as her next target. Her list of targets for Special Times was: 'pausing; speaking slower; repeating back what Khaled says.'

Family strategy reviewed: 'Building my child's confidence'

Family strategy reviewed: 'Bedtimes'

Family strategy discussed: 'Behaviour management'

Session 6

Session 6 of Palin PCI therapy begins with the same format as the previous sessions (see below). We then discuss the consolidation period, and arrange an appointment for the review.

- Review of Special Times and task sheets
- Record the interaction video
- Watch the video and review the target or introduce a new target
- Set Special Times targets and give task sheets
- Make another video recording if necessary
- Discuss the family strategy
- Discuss the consolidation period (see below)
- Arrange the review appointment.

A review appointment is booked in six weeks' time, when the parents will return with the child.

Case study *Scott, aged three years*

Session 6

Both Scott's parents had completed their Special Times and brought in their task sheets. A video recording was made and Scott's father noticed that he was pausing and talking slowly throughout the play session, and that Scott did not stammer once on the video. He said that it was becoming much easier to 'switch into slow mode' and he found himself doing it quite often when he was talking to Scott. His mother was also pleased with her video: she felt that she was giving him plenty of time to think of and say what he wanted, and she thought that she seemed more focused on him, rather than on what she was doing or thinking. Both parents decided that they would maintain their targets on an ongoing basis, as well as also trying to use them when they remembered outside of Special Times.

Family strategy reviewed: 'Building my child's confidence'

Family strategy reviewed: 'Turn-taking'

Family strategies discussed: 'Feelings' and 'The child whose standards are too high'

Case study *Khaled, aged five years*

Session 6

Khaled's mother had done her Special Times and recorded on her sheet that it was 'not really an effort to do it this way any more.' She also found it quite easy to do more repetition of what Khaled was saying. She reported that she was using the pausing and slower rate often with both boys, except when life 'got a bit out of hand.' She was praised for doing this and reassured that nobody can remain calm all the time! It was agreed that she would maintain the three targets in her Special Times over the next six weeks during the consolidation period and return her task sheets.

Family strategy reviewed: 'Building my child's confidence'

Family strategy reviewed: 'Bedtimes'

Family strategy reviewed: 'Behaviour management'

Summary of Sessions 1 to 6

During the initial six weeks of therapy, we set up Special Times and introduce up to three interaction targets. We introduce the family strategy of 'Building my child's confidence' and any other relevant topics. We review and collect the parents' task sheets.

The consolidation period

The consolidation period is six weeks of parent-led, home-based therapy. We remind parents that it is during the consolidation period that fluency improvement is expected. We tell the parents that if there is any deterioration in the child's fluency during this time, they should telephone us to discuss this.

During this six-week phase of Palin PCI the family does not attend the clinic but continues to implement the treatment plan at home with the child. Special Times continue with the same targets and the same frequency. The parents complete their task sheets and send them to us at the end of each week. They continue to praise their child daily and send in the 'Praise log' weekly (as described in Chapter 7). During this period they also maintain the other family strategies that have been discussed.

The parents send in the task sheets and 'Praise logs', and we make contact with them to provide positive feedback, or if forms are not received or if problems have arisen. Parents are encouraged to contact us if they have any concerns about their tasks or the child's progress.

In our clinical experience, improvement in the child's stammering tends to occur during the initial six weeks of Palin PCI or in the consolidation period, and may continue for a number of months after this. This is supported by our research evidence (Millard *et al*, 2008).

If parents report that the child's stammering has become worse, we explore possible reasons for the deterioration, for example whether the child or another family member has been ill, tiredness, unusual levels of excitement, disruption to the usual family routine, an incident at home or school. We often find that Special Times are no longer in place, especially if there has been a disruption to the child's or family's lifestyle. Parents may need help in reinstating Special Times and their targets, in praising their child and in any other relevant family strategies. If we cannot identify a possible explanation for the deterioration in the child's speech, we encourage parents to continue with their tasks until the review appointment, when we make further management decisions.

Case study *Scott, aged three years*

Scott's parents sent in their task sheets and 'Praise logs' for the first three weeks, in which they recorded that Special Times and 'Praise' were going well. They had noticed that throughout the day they were conscious of helping Scott to give himself more time. They did not send in any sheets at the end of the fourth week and when contact was made they said that Scott's mother had had to go into hospital and everything was in turmoil, and Scott's stammering had been a lot worse. She was now home and both parents had reinstated Special Times and the other family strategies, and Scott's stammering had settled down again. They continued to send in their sheets for the last two weeks.

Case study *Khaled, aged five years*

Khaled's mother did not send her sheets in at the end of the first week. When she was contacted she said that she had been doing her Special Times and the other tasks, but she had not written them down. The reasons for writing and sending her task sheets were discussed and she was happy to complete the sheets in future. She then returned the sheets for the remainder of the consolidation period.

The review appointment

At the end of the six-week consolidation period the parents bring the child to the clinic to discuss his progress and agree future input.

Reassessment

- *Parental report:* we ask the parents to rate their child's level of stammering using the same severity rating scale used in the case history. We also ask them to rate their level of concern about the child's speech on the rating scale (see Chapter 4). If the child is still stammering, we ask the parents to describe the nature of the stammering. This enables us to monitor any qualitative changes in the child's speech.
- *Assessment:* we also obtain a speech sample using the *'What's Wrong?'* pictures (LDA, 1988). This is audio- or video-recorded, transcribed and analysed as in the initial child assessment (see Chapter 4). We then compare the percentage of stammering with the levels before treatment, as well as any qualitative changes in the stammering. We also ask the child how he is getting on with his speech.

Clinical decision-making

- *Improvement:* if both parental report and the assessment indicate that the child's speech is improving and parental anxiety is decreasing, we encourage the parents to continue with the regimen of Special Times, praise and other family strategies. Sometimes parents find it harder to keep up these tasks when they are less concerned about the child's speech. We point out that the child's fluency remains vulnerable and that the parents will need to keep up these strategies.
- *Stammering persists:* if the child's stammering has not improved we may arrange further sessions to work on interaction strategies or family strategies. This may be because new issues have emerged, or there may be strategies which were identified in the full assessment which were not covered in the first six sessions of therapy. If the identified interaction and family strategies are already in place and the child's fluency remains a cause for concern, some kind of direct therapy can be used. This is discussed further in Chapter 8.

Case study *Scott, aged three years*

Review appointment

At the review appointment, Scott's parents reported that they were very pleased with his progress: he was stammering much less now. When he was reassessed his percentage of stammered syllables was 1.6 per cent and his stammering featured part-word repetitions only. His mother rated his severity at 2 and his father at 1 on the severity rating scale. They both rated their level of concern as 1. They felt that the programme of confidence-building had been very helpful, and they both found it 'second nature' to use the specific praise model. They were also trying to encourage him to express his feelings using strategies from the handout, and Scott's mother said she was trying hard to be 'a model of imperfection' to help Scott lower his extremely high standards. Turn-taking was still a challenge with the twins, but they still remembered the Microphone Game and waving an imaginary magic wand. The family were encouraged to continue with the Special Times and the family strategies, and they decided that it would be helpful to continue to send their sheets in for the next three months. They were advised to contact the therapist if they became concerned about Scott's speech, but they said that they felt that even if he did have a setback, they would know how to help him.

Case study *Khaled, aged five years*

Review appointment

Khaled's mother reported that he was stammering less and she rated the severity as 2 and her concern about it also as 2. In the reassessment, Khaled stammered on three per cent of syllables spoken and his stammering featured repetitions of whole words and parts of words. His mother was delighted with his progress and felt that his fluency was much better now that he was not so tired and because she was helping him to take his time. She was also very pleased with her ability to manage his behaviour. She said that she still thought he talked a bit too fast, even when she was talking more slowly to him, and his speech was still difficult for others to understand, owing to the speech sound substitutions. It was agreed that a block of six sessions would be arranged to address some of these concerns. Meanwhile, Khaled's mother would continue to do Special Times, complete and send in the sheets, and implement the family strategies.

See Chapter 8 for further details of Khaled's management.

Ongoing monitoring

We continue to monitor the child's progress for a period of at least one year. We would normally arrange further review appointments at three months, six months and one year after the review session. We encourage the parents to contact us at any point if they are concerned about their child's speech.

> ***Case study*** *Scott, aged three years*
>
> *Scott's parents attended review appointments at three, six and 12 months. He had suffered minor lapses in his fluency, once when he was ill and then over the Christmas period. His parents had continued to do the Special Times and at the one-year review they were no longer concerned about his speech; they said that he hardly ever stammered and even when he did it sounded like normal hesitation. We assured Scott's parents that they could contact us at any stage in the future. We did not hear from them again, so we contacted them three years later and Scott's mother told us that he was fine now and they had almost forgotten he had ever had a problem with his speech.*
>
> *In total Scott attended for the full assessment, six therapy sessions and four review sessions.*

Discharge

At the one-year review, if parents are no longer concerned about their child's speech, we would normally discuss discharging the child. However, over the years we have seen some children, whose fluency appears to have resolved completely, return to the clinic several years later because there has been a relapse. We therefore explain to parents that we will be discharging their child, but, if at any point in the future they should become concerned about the child's fluency, they should not hesitate to contact us. Thus we maintain an 'open door' policy to take account of the unpredictable nature of stammering and the possibility of relapse.

Specialist advice

Stammering is a complex disorder, and some children who stammer present with additional complications. These may take the form of coexisting difficulties, such as specific language impairment, Down's syndrome or dyspraxia. For some children who stammer there may be concerns about psychological factors, such as anxiety or selective mutism. Alternatively, there may be family problems such as relationship difficulties or major health issues.

When there are added complexities such as those suggested, or when progress in therapy is not as expected, we recommend that therapists seek specialist advice. There may be a specialist SLT for stammering who is available to provide support. The MPC offers telephone or email advice to SLTs from the UK and beyond. Furthermore, at the MPC we offer charitably funded consultation clinics for children who live in the UK. We accept referrals from SLTs, who are invited to attend the assessment with the family. Two MPC therapists are involved in the consultation. One assesses the child while the other does a detailed parent interview with both parents, which the referring therapist observes. Once the information has been gathered, the MPC therapists develop a formulation and discuss therapy recommendations with the referring therapist. When this has been agreed, the formulation and recommendations are presented to the parents. A clinical report is then written and the therapist is encouraged to maintain a close liaison with the MPC, seeking further support or advice as necessary. A review appointment is then offered to the family and referring therapist six months later, when progress can be discussed and further recommendations made, in consultation with the referring SLT. This consultation is free of charge to the family and the SLT. If the case is particularly complex and the referring therapist feels that she does not have the skills required to provide the therapy, we sometimes offer therapy to the family at the MPC, with funding being sought from the family's local primary care trust.

Troubleshooting

The child wants his parents' attention and makes it difficult for them to watch the video in the session

Typically, we have found that children either enjoy watching the video of themselves playing, or they are happy to carry on with the play activity that they have started with their parents. If the child is bored with that activity we encourage him to choose something different, checking that it is something that he can do on his own. If there are two parents, we sometimes ask one parent to play with the child while we watch and discuss the video with the other. If we are working with one parent, we might negotiate with the child that if he can let his parent talk to us for 10 minutes, he will then have an extra playtime afterwards. It may be helpful to set up a star chart with the child, rewarding him for waiting while the adults finish their conversation. (For details on how to set up a star chart, see Chapter 7.)

The parent chooses a target which is different from the one(s) that the therapist has identified

In the original analysis of the parent–child interaction we identify which interaction styles the child needs to build his fluency, when the parent is using these and which ones could be developed further. Thus, at the beginning of therapy we have in mind a number of interaction styles which might help the child. However, we let the parents identify their own targets and sometimes they focus on a different target. In our experience this is not a problem. Interaction styles are very closely linked together and making a change to one aspect often has a 'ripple' effect on many others. For example, if a parent decides to sit back a bit more and let the child take charge, this often results in the parent giving the child more time to speak, using more commenting and using language which is at the child's level. We have also found that parents may use different terms of reference to us. For example, Scott's father described Scott's need for pausing and thinking time as 'he needs to digest in his head'.

One parent is achieving his target and moving on to a new one, whereas the other parent is still on the first target

We do not expect two parents to move through therapy at the same pace and we sometimes find that one parent has the same target for the six weeks. We would gently and humorously discourage any spirit of competition between parents, and we suggest that it is helpful that the parent is ensuring that the target is fully assimilated before moving on.

Parents not used to playing with child

We have worked with some parents who have had very little experience of playing with their child, for a variety of cultural and social reasons. However, this does not usually mean that the child does not know how to play and sometimes we can help them to see that they just need to take their cue from the child. Some parents feel that they should always take the opportunity to teach the child. We have usually found that watching themselves on the video helps the parents to engage more in the play. Many play activities mimic real life, for example play kitchen and food, medical kits, car, road and garage sets. Parents who are not used to imaginary play may find it easier to become engaged with these toys.

No video camera

A video camera is an invaluable tool for an SLT in the assessment and management of a wide range of disorders. Parent–child interaction therapy is widely used in the management of other speech and language problems. Making video recordings of our own clinical practice is also very useful in reflective practice and supervision. If the SLT does not have a video, we recommend that a request is made to purchase one, and good quality cameras are now available at a reasonable cost. If equipment cannot be purchased, it is possible that the SLT service may have one available for loan, or some clinics have systems available for their staff. Alternatively, it is possible that the family you are working with has their own camera, which could be used in the sessions.

Only one parent arrives for session

If therapy sessions have been arranged for both parents and only one parent arrives for an appointment it is important, firstly, to find out why the other parent has not come. If it seems that a parent is unsure about the necessity of their involvement, we have a conversation about the benefits of both parents being involved in the process. We need to be sensitive to the fact that the parent who is present is not likely to be the one who is questioning this process, and we might be putting them in a difficult position. We may decide to do the therapy session with the parent who has come or we may reschedule the appointment. We ask them to telephone in future if one of them will be unable to come, so that we can rearrange the appointment to suit them both. If necessary we may telephone the other parent to discuss any queries they may have about their role in therapy.

Parent cannot answer questions, especially about self on video, and wants SLT to tell them the answers

We have occasionally found that a parent finds it difficult to answer the questions about the video. In our experience this has not been related to their level of insight or understanding about their child. It is more likely to be because they think that we are looking for a certain answer and they are worried they might be 'wrong'. Sometimes parents expect the 'expert' to tell them. As we discussed at the beginning of this chapter, we have found that eliciting this information from parents is more effective than telling them, but, if they find this process frustrating or stressful, we help them by showing specific video clips and giving hints, and ultimately giving them the information if necessary.

When the parent starts doing a second target, he stops doing the first

Making a change to our habitual style is a challenge. Making two changes may be too difficult, especially if the first change is not fully consolidated. We need to monitor carefully that the parent has integrated their first target into their interaction style, before introducing any further changes.

Parents uncomfortable about talking about their child while he is present

Parents may feel inhibited about talking about their child in front of him, especially if the child tends to listen and has well-developed comprehension. If the topic of conversation is a sensitive one, we might arrange a separate appointment for the parents to attend without the child.

Special Times issues

A parent has been unable to do as many Special Times as agreed

When a five-minute task is suggested, most people think it is easily achievable. However, busy lifestyles and unexpected events may scupper the best of intentions. We help the parents by asking, 'What got in the way of you doing your Special Times?' Together, we can explore potential solutions. Sometimes parents need to reduce the target number of Special Times, for example if they initially chose to do five, it might be more realistic to change this to three.

If a parent has not managed to do the minimum of three Special Times, we set the task for a second week without any interaction targets being incorporated. If one parent has completed the target number of Special Times, but the other parent has not, we reset the task for both parents. It is essential that the parents establish the routine of Special Times before therapy moves forward.

In some cases, it may be a difficult time for the parents to be starting Palin PCI, especially if there are other stresses. In some situations it may be better to delay therapy until the parents feel they can give it their best shot.

The Special Times lasted longer than five minutes

It can be difficult to keep to five minutes, especially if the activity is unfinished. We ask the parents what they think are the reasons for the five-minute time limit and we suggest that the activities should not be too complicated. We sometimes suggest the use of a timer and reiterate that they can go back to the activity once they have completed the task sheet.

For some parents, limiting the time in Special Times may be an important step in setting some boundaries for their child.

The child did not want to do the Special Times

This rarely occurs, but if parents are reporting that the child does not want do Special Times it may be worth checking who is choosing the activity, as well as how and when the child is being asked to play. It is possible that the parent is suggesting a Special Time when the child is doing something he particularly enjoys, for example watching a favourite television programme. We sometimes remind the child that he agreed to help his parents with their homework.

The parent has made a record of the child's fluency

We remind parents to use the Special Times to focus on having fun and listening to what the child is saying, rather than how he is saying it.

The parent is doing the Special Times while doing something else

Busy schedules may result in parents incorporating Special Times into other activities, for example bath time, homework, journeys. In such cases we explore with the parents why this is not ideal: for example, the child is less likely to have his parents' undivided attention, there may be interruptions from others or the focus is not on the child.

A sibling is interrupting the Special Times

Parents may report that their child's sibling is interrupting the Special Times. We discuss with them how they think this could be tackled, checking whether they are also giving the sibling Special Times, as suggested. We may recommend that they have a conversation with the children about taking turns with Special Times and deciding who will go first. We may also explore where and when the Special Times are happening and whether changing this might make interruptions less likely. Sometimes it is helpful to do Special Times when siblings are otherwise occupied, for example asleep!

Rationale for interaction targets

The rationale is important for parents

During Palin PCI sessions, once the parents have identified an interaction target to focus on, we encourage them to think about why that interaction target may be helpful for a child's fluency. Therapists will need to know how and why different interaction strategies enhance a child's fluency.

Listed below is the range of interaction targets focused on during therapy, along with the evidence to support their potential inclusion in an individualised therapy programme. Although some of the interaction targets have been researched in relation to their impact on stammering, other targets are based on clinical expertise and experience of what helps a child be more fluent.

We also present what is involved in achieving each interaction target and a description of how each target may play a role in facilitating fluency. We also consider each target in relation to its potential impact on facilitating a child's language development. This is because some CWS also present with other speech and language difficulties and there are a number of similarities between Palin PCI and other parent-focused interventions for children with language impairment (Girolametto *et al*, 1986; Manolson, 1992; Weistuch *et al*, 1991).

Palin PCI rule of thumb:
The child needs to give himself time to plan and execute what he wants to say, at a pace and a level that will support his fluency

The overall aim of each target is to ensure that a child gives himself time to plan and execute what he wants to say and is able to function at an appropriate level given his abilities.

Following the child's lead in play

What is involved?

We have found this to be one of the key interaction targets identified by parents as supporting their child's fluency. 'Following the child's lead in play' is a broad term which encompasses a number of different interaction targets. It involves parents:

- Watching what the child is doing, rather than initiating and playing with the toys themselves
- Commenting on and responding to what the child is interested in, or is focused on, rather than asking questions or giving instructions
- Allowing the child to solve problems for himself
- Joining in with the child's chosen activity and copying what the child is doing.

A parent may select one of the above targets to focus on when working on following their child's lead and then build on it over subsequent sessions.

Support for this target

We have noticed that if a parent follows the child's lead in play, the pace of the play is more likely to progress at a child's natural level rather than that of the parent. The child will therefore have more time to plan and initiate what he wants to say.

Andronico and Blake (1971) found the fluency of children who stammered was increased when their parents were trained in non-directive play sessions. If the parent is following the child's lead, they are more likely to have a joint focus of attention, which has been found to promote vocabulary development (Smith *et al*, 1988; Tomasello & Todd, 1983) and more frequent and longer conversations (Tomasello & Farrar, 1986).

Letting the child solve problems for himself

What is involved?

We know that children tend to vary in their response to problems in play, such as having difficulty putting together two pieces of Lego ® or managing something getting stuck. Some children are keen to work things out for themselves, whereas others quickly become frustrated and demand help. In order for parents to let the child solve the problem for himself, they will need to:

- Watch and wait – giving the child time to solve the problem for himself
- Acknowledge the problem
- Encourage the child in his attempts to solve it
- Offer support if needed.

Support for this target

We have found that encouraging parents to give their child more time to work out problems can be helpful in a number of ways:

- It contributes to the overall pace of play being at the child's level
- It encourages a child's problem-solving skills
- It increases a child's self-confidence.

Using more comments than questions during conversation

What is involved?

Although questions are a typical feature of any interaction, we have found that it may be helpful for the child if a parent uses more comments than questions during play. Commenting does not demand a response, although the child may choose to reply. If a child is quiet, a natural reaction is to attempt to engage him by asking a question.

In order for parents to use more comments than questions during play, they will need to:

- Understand the difference between comments and questions
- Learn how to change a question into a comment
- Make more comments
- Ask fewer questions.

Support for this target

The use of commenting may be as effective as asking questions in generating conversation without demands being placed on the child's language skills or fluency. When parents comment during play, they can introduce vocabulary and language structures which are relevant to what the child is doing. This joint focus of attention facilitates language development (Girolametto *et al*, 2000; Tomasello & Todd, 1983) and demonstrates to the child that his parent is interested and involved in the activity.

Complexity of questions at child's level

What is involved?

Parents will need to:

- Understand the child's language level
- Understand that different questions have varying levels of complexity.

Support for this target

Although research has not found that children are more likely to stammer when answering questions (Weiss & Zebrowski, 1992; Wilkenfeld & Curlee, 1997; Bernstein Ratner, 2001), it has been suggested that parents may help their child's fluency by considering the types of questions they tend to use, as a child is more likely to stammer when answering questions that require a longer or more complex answer.

Different question forms require varying levels of complexity in their response. Questions may range from requiring a simple one-word answer to a request for complex information:

- 'Yes/No'
- Forced alternatives
- 'What?'

- 'When?'
- 'Why/How?'
- Open-ended questions, such as 'Tell me about…?'

We have found it helpful to tailor the level of complexity of questions to the child's ability to understand and to formulate a matching response.

Using language which is appropriate for the child's level

What is involved?

We have found that it is helpful for some children when parents are aware of the language they use and focus on talking at a level of input that is within the child's range of linguistic competence.

Parents will need to:

- Understand their child's language level
- Be aware of their own language level
- Fine-tune their input to that of their child.

Support for this target

Research tells us that although there is individual variation, a child is more likely to stammer when he uses sentences that are longer and more complex (Bernstein Ratner & Sih, 1987; Gaines *et al*, 1991; Logan & Conture, 1995, 1997; Weiss & Zebrowski, 1992; Yaruss, 1999). It has also been found that if a child is talking at a level that is within his range of linguistic competence he is making it easier for himself to be fluent (Bernstein Ratner, 1997a; Zackheim & Conture, 2003).

Whilst some studies have found no differences between parents of CWS and parents of fluent children in terms of the complexity of the language they use when speaking to their children (Kloth *et al*, 1995b, 1998; Yaruss & Conture, 1995; Miles & Bernstein Ratner, 2001), other studies have associated the use of longer, more complex parental language with persistence (Kloth *et al*, 1999; Rommel *et al*, 1999; Rommel, 2000).

This target may be particularly important for those children who also have delayed language development. The use of language that is slightly more advanced than the child's ability has been found to be helpful in encouraging the development of language in young children (Yoder & Warren, 1993).

Studies looking at fathers' interaction styles have found that, in general, fathers tend to use more complex language and a more sophisticated vocabulary when interacting with their children than mothers (Conti-Ramsden *et al*,

1995). Similar findings have been reported in studies of children who stammer and their fathers (Kelly, 1994b, 1995). It may therefore be particularly helpful to observe a father's language level.

There has been some concern expressed in the literature that use of simplified language as a fluency-enhancing strategy may have a negative effect on a child's language development, in particular for those CWS who also present with delayed speech and language skills (Miles & Bernstein Ratner, 2001; Ratner & Silverman, 2000). A study to investigate the impact of Palin PCI on children's language development showed that the group of children included in the study continued to develop language over the period they were receiving Palin PCI and for a period of time after therapy. There was therefore no evidence that Palin PCI impedes language development in CWS (Nicholas *et al*, 2004).

Using language which is semantically contingent on the child's focus of attention

What is involved?

Parents will need to:

- Watch the child's activity
- Talk to the child about what he is doing
- Listen to the child
- Respond to the child's conversational topic.

Support for this target

We have found that if parents talk to the child about what is taking place in the 'here and now', this will help the child to understand what is being said, as well as helping him to respond using language which is relevant to the play. Talking about something which is not in the 'here and now' is more linguistically challenging and this might affect a child's ability to be fluent, especially if he has restricted language skills.

Using repetition, expansion and rephrasing of the child's utterance

What is involved?

Parents will need to:

- Listen carefully to what the child is saying
- Learn how to expand to an appropriate level
- Use repetition and rephrasing as required.

Support for this target

Repetition, expansion and rephrasing are generally useful strategies in facilitating young children's language development (Girolametto *et al*, 1999; Nelson *et al*, 1996). Repetition is also helpful if a child's speech is unclear as it provides a clear model and allows the parent to check with the child that they have understood. We would therefore predict that these styles may also facilitate a child's fluency if the child has restricted speech and language skills.

Giving the child time to initiate, respond and finish his talking

What is involved?

Parents will need to:

- Allow silences to happen
- Use longer pauses before speaking and between utterances
- Listen to the child and ensure that he has finished speaking before the parent speaks again.

Support for this target

- *Time to initiate:* given that CWS may need to allow more time to plan and organise what they want to say, it follows that giving a child time to initiate language during play may be helpful for his fluency. Parents tell us that they have to learn to tolerate lengthier pauses, and not be tempted to fill silences with a question or comment.
- *Time to respond:* a child whose fluency is vulnerable may benefit from being allowed a longer time to respond, particularly when a longer or more complex response is required. Newman and Smit (1989) found that if an adult waited for longer before responding to a child, the child would also increase his response time. They also found that three of the four children in their study stammered less when the adult's response time latency was longer.
- *Time to finish his talking:* we have found that it is more helpful when parents wait until the child has finished talking before they respond rather than interrupting or finishing the sentence for him.

Research has shown that stammering influences parents' interaction styles, in particular their interrupting behaviours. Mothers of both CWS and fluent children were more likely to interrupt when a child spoke dysfluently than when they spoke fluently (Meyers & Freeman, 1985a). In addition, mothers were more likely to interrupt or talk at the same time as their child the more severe a child's stammering (Kelly & Conture, 1992). Among their interpretation of the findings, Kelly and Conture (1992) suggested that mothers may, consciously or unconsciously, think they are helping their child by interrupting and finishing off their sentences for them.

Winslow and Guitar (1994) demonstrated that it is helpful for parents to be aware of family turn-taking patterns. They asked a five-year-old boy and his family to carry out a structured conversational turn-taking routine during mealtimes over a seven-week period, where interruptions were discouraged and appropriate turn-taking behaviour was praised. The child's stammering was found to be less during the sessions where turn-taking rules were used.

Matching the parent's rate to the child's rate of speech

What is involved?

A parent will need to:

- Listen to the child's rate of speech
- Listen to their own rate of speech
- Try to match their rate to the child's
- Try to maintain naturalness and normal intonation patterns.

Support for this target

Some research has found that parents can help their child's fluency by speaking more slowly (Guitar & Marchinkoski, 2001; Guitar *et al*, 1992; Stephenson-Opsal & Bernstein Ratner 1988; Zebrowski *et al*, 1996). However, it is not yet clear how a slower parental rate facilitates a child's fluency. It might be predicted that parents modelling a slower rate would result in a corresponding reduction in the children's rate. The research has not found this to be the case (Bernstein Ratner 1992; Stephenson-Opsal & Bernstein Ratner, 1988). When mothers were asked to speak more slowly, Bernstein Ratner (1992) found that they also spoke using shorter and less complex sentences, and they had longer pauses between turns. It may therefore be these features of a parent's interaction style which are important in facilitating fluency rather than just slowing down.

A slower parental rate may also be helpful for those children with language difficulties. Children with specific language impairment have been found to benefit from having material presented to them at a slower pace (Montgomery, 2005).

When considering their own rate, parents often want to know how slowly they should be going. The research would suggest that parents can help their children's fluency by comparing their rate with their child's rate. Yaruss and Conture (1995) found that the greater the difference between a mother's and a child's rate, the more severe the child's stammer. We therefore help parents to speak at a rate which is similar to, or slightly slower than, their child's rate. Although parents are speaking more slowly, they are encouraged to sound as natural as possible, to use appropriate intonation and not to become 'choppy' or sound like a 'robot'. Video feedback can help parents to achieve a slower rate that they like the sound of.

Using pausing before and between utterances

What is involved?

Parents will need to:

- Increase their use of pausing between sentences
- Increase their use of pausing between turns.

Support for this target

This may be helpful in a number of ways:

- It slows down the overall pace of the interaction
- The parent's pause provides time for the child to plan and execute his response
- It provides a model for the child to use more pausing. If the child uses pausing, he allows himself more time, which, in turn, may facilitate his fluency.

Use of eye contact, position, touch, humour and/or surprise

What is involved?

A parent will need to:

- Be aware of their position
- Be aware of their own use of eye contact
- Make changes as appropriate
- Experiment with touch and humour and/or surprise.

Support for target

Clinical experience has shown that parents may need to help their child to develop their use of eye contact. Making eye contact with a child may help him to focus on the activity and what he is saying, which, in turn, may help his fluency. Positioning can facilitate eye contact – being at the same level as the child, with appropriate proximity and face-to-face.

Some children find it difficult to maintain concentration on an activity when there are visual or auditory distractions. Others may be single-channelled in their attention, finding it difficult to talk while they are focused on an activity. Parents may need to help these children by the use of a number of strategies to gain or maintain their concentration, including touch, surprise and humour.

Using praise and reinforcement

What is involved?

A parent will need to:

- Observe what the child is doing
- Identify opportunities for praise
- Explore suitable language for praise.

Support for this target

Praise and reinforcement may be helpful for the child who stammers, in encouraging motivation, developing their individual potential, promoting independence and autonomy (Henderlong & Lepper, 2002) and encouraging confidence, all of which could be considered essential for developing social communication skills.

7

Family Strategies

In the full assessment, the parents may have identified a number of areas that they feel have an effect on the child's daily life and therefore his fluency. Most of these issues are common parenting challenges, and we do not consider them to be causing the stammering. However, if parents raise these as areas of concern we want to offer support or, if appropriate, help them to find an alternative source of help. Therapists may have some concerns about addressing parenting issues, so in this chapter we will present some simple ideas to guide therapists as they help the parents to make small changes to their management which might affect the child's fluency. We do not consider ourselves to be 'gurus' of child-rearing. We will leave that to other experts.

Family strategies:
- *Special Times*
- *Managing two languages*
- *Openness about stammering*
- *Building confidence*
- *Turn-taking*
- *Dealing with feelings*
- *High standards*
- *Sleep*
- *Behaviour management*
- *Routines*
- *Pace of life*
- *Emerging issues*

In the sections that follow we describe techniques and approaches which we have used with families. In some sections we have included interactive handouts for parents, which we would usually give them to read and complete the week before we plan to discuss the topic. This enables parents to think about the issues and how they affect their child, as well as to consider some practical ideas to help them. We have found that parents may agree or disagree with what is written and this stimulates them to explore the topic with us. Sometimes parents come to the session having already tried out some of the suggestions.

After the full assessment, we have identified which family strategies are to be included in the therapy programme and each strategy has been ticked on the Summary Chart (see Appendix III).

The first family strategy to be introduced is 'Special Times', which was described in Chapter 6 and is an integral part of the therapy programme for all families.

If needed, we also discuss the family strategy 'Managing two languages', in the first or second session.

If the parents are finding it difficult to be open about their child's stammer, we would give them the handout for the family strategy 'Openness about stammering' (see Appendix XXII) in the first session for them to read and discuss with us in the second session.

'Building my child's confidence' is an integral family strategy within the therapy programme, and we typically give parents the handout (see Appendix XXI) for this in the third therapy session and we discuss it in the fourth session.

After this, we cover topics as appropriate and we may ask parents to prioritise them if there are several.

We sometimes find that new issues arise during the course of therapy or at a later stage, for example if the child starts at school or preschool or if there is a family bereavement. The 'Emerging issues' section (p.165) covers the issues we sometimes have encountered.

It is important that, as therapists, we receive our own support and supervision as advised by our professional bodies, particularly if we are developing new skills or working with sensitive issues. This helps our professional development, but also enables us to recognise the limits of our own expertise so that we make responsible decisions about onward referral.

Special Times

This family strategy is described in Chapter 6 and is included in the therapy programme for all families.

Managing two languages

Many children grow up in households where two or more languages are spoken and a proportion of these children will stammer. Learning more than one language may place an extra demand on some children's fluency and we may need to help parents find ways of managing this.

Helping the parents to manage two languages

We discuss with the parents their feelings about their child's ability to manage two or more languages and give information and advice as follows.

Bilingualism does not cause stammering

During the full assessment some parents express their concern that the child is stammering because the family is using two or more languages. In the formulation (see Chapter 5) we use the multifactorial model to allay their fears that it has caused the problem.

In the therapy session we can remind parents of the range of factors which may be relevant in the development of the child's stammer in order to reinforce the fact that the child's language environment is not the reason why the child started to stammer.

We can tell parents that bilingual children often have a surge in language at around three years of age. It is possible that this surge may occur when the child's stammering first emerged, as his linguistic abilities might have been outstripping his speech motor skills.

- *Bilingualism does not cause stammering*
- *Code-switching is fine*
- *Consistency might help*

Code-switching is fine

Bilingual speakers often mix two languages as they speak. Code-switching is a natural phenomenon because people often use the word that they think of first, whether it be their home language or English.

Whereas once it was thought that this might make it more difficult for the child who stammers, we would now encourage parents to speak to their child in the way which is most comfortable for them. This will preserve the quality and naturalness of the parent–child communication, giving the child a rich and full language model.

Consistency might help some children

If we feel that the child is struggling to process more than one language and this is affecting his fluency, we may help the parents to decide how to build in some consistency in the child's language environment, for example:

- The parents will speak their home language and the school staff will use English
- The grandparents will use their home language, everybody else will use English
- The mother will use English, the father will use his home language.

In this way, the child will know what language to expect.

Case study *Khaled, aged five years*

Session 1

Khaled's mother was reassured that the family's use of Arabic had not caused his stammering. The therapist pointed out that his understanding and use of English were age-appropriate. Khaled's mother asked if she should stop using Arabic and she was advised that this was not necessary, as he seemed to be coping well with both languages. She said that she tended to mix the languages and she was reminded that this was fine, as it would give Khaled a natural and rich language model.

Openness about stammering

How parents respond

Listening to a child stammering can be difficult. People may experience feelings of distress, pity, anxiety, shock, panic, frustration or bewilderment. For the parents of that child, these emotions can be very strong (Zebrowski & Schum, 1993) and they may be compounded when a parent has or has had a stammer themselves. If, as is commonly the case, the child has started to speak fluently but then gradually or suddenly 'loses' this fluency, parents may find this more traumatic. Many parents are therefore likely to be experiencing very upsetting thoughts and emotions as they listen to their child struggling to speak fluently, and naturally they may be unsure as to how they should respond.

The conspiracy of silence

The field of stammering therapy has had a chequered history when it comes to advising parents on how to react when their child is stammering. Very early theories (Johnson, 1942) implied that it would be damaging to the child if his attention were drawn to his stumblings and hesitations when speaking. Parents were told not to react in any way to stammering, to mask their anxieties and fears, to listen and respond as if nothing were wrong. Presumably, a child who was highly aware of his stammering would have been mystified by this response, perhaps deducing that there existed some taboo about his talking, that it was somehow unmentionable. It is possible that this may account for the number of adults who stammer who now report that they have never talked to anyone about their difficulty and who have made every effort to disguise or hide it.

It is fine to acknowledge it

There has been a misperception that indirect approaches to early stammering perpetuated this 'conspiracy of silence'. On the contrary, early publications about parent–child interaction therapy advocated that stammering should be openly acknowledged and discussed. In 1991, Botterill *et al* advised that parents keep an open dialogue with the child about stammering. Other therapy approaches, such as the Lidcombe Program (Onslow *et al*, 2003), also encourage parents to be open about their child's stammering, giving structured feedback to develop the child's fluency.

Helping parents to be open about stammering

If the full assessment has indicated that the family has been unsure about whether or how to talk to the child about his stammering, this issue is discussed early in the therapy programme.

Handout:
Openness about stammering

Handout

At the end of the first therapy session we give each parent the handout, 'Openness about stammering' (see Appendix XXII). We ask them to read it at home, answer the questions and consider the suggestions, then bring it with them to the next session.

Feedback

In the second session we ask them what they thought about the handout and look at what they have written.

Discussion: Why is it helpful to be open?

We start by discussing with the parents the reasons for being open about the stammering with the child. We might ask:

- 'Why might it help your child when you talk to him about his stammering?'
- 'What might the child think if he realises he has a problem talking, but nobody else ever mentions it?'

We suggest that when a parent notices the child's struggles and sympathises with him, they potentially open up a dialogue about the stammering, which the child can choose to enter or not. This is especially appropriate for the child who is aware that he is stammering. He has been given a signal that it is acceptable to talk about his difficulty, rather than pretending it is not there. Acknowledging it in a relaxed and natural way may help the child to feel less anxious about what is happening to his speech, which may in turn improve his fluency.

Brainstorm: what to say?

On the handout (Appendix XXII), the parents have recorded how they respond when their child is struggling with anything. We use this to help them think of the way they could talk to him about his stammering, and brainstorm a range of possible responses:

- 'Oh that was hard to say, wasn't it?'
- 'That was a struggle – well done, you got there!'
- 'Those words were tricky.'
- 'Sometimes it's hard to talk, isn't it?'

We ask the parents which phrases they would be comfortable using with their child. Sometimes children acknowledge their parents' comments about their stammering, but if the child does not react, we would still encourage the parent to be open about the stammering.

Discussion: how parents can help their child to see that we all make mistakes

As well as acknowledging a child's stammering, we also encourage parents to notice their own stumblings and hesitations and make comments on their own fluency:

- 'Do you know, today I don't seem to be able to string a sentence together'
- 'My words seem to be getting stuck at the moment'
- 'That didn't come out right, did it?'
- 'I can't get my tongue around that word'.

The child is helped to see that lots of people make 'mistakes' when they speak. A child who is very sensitive to his own mistakes may set himself slightly lower standards if he learns that everybody is dysfluent sometimes. Not only will this help reassure the child, it will also help parents to adjust their expectations of 'normal' fluency as they focus on their own fluency and that of others who do not stammer.

Giving advice about stammering

Parents may be tempted to acknowledge their child's stammer by giving advice such as 'slow down', 'stop and start again', 'take a breath' and so on. Although such comments can be helpful to some children, we typically advise parents to err on the side of caution on the amount of advice they give their child. A child can interpret such advice as getting their speech wrong. They then try hard to be more fluent, which may make things worse. If parents feel they want to do something, we often suggest that they think about their own speech first before commenting on the child's. At these early stages of stammering it may be more helpful if they model a slower rate with frequent pauses, rather than asking the child to slow down. This may encourage the child to take his time and make use of pauses too. It also helps parents to discover how hard it is to follow such advice.

Case study *Scott, aged three years*

Session 1

Scott's parents were each given a copy of the handout 'Openness about stammering' (see Appendix XXII) and asked to read it, answer any questions and consider the ideas suggested.

Session 2

The handout was discussed and both Scott's parents said that they felt better about acknowledging his stammer, as they could see that it would make him feel it was OK to talk about it. They thought he might even keep trying when he stammered, rather than give up, as he had started to do. They said that they had already started to make the occasional comment when Scott really struggled and he had seemed fine about it.

Session 3

Scott's parents commented that they now found it very natural and 'quite a relief' to make a comment when they noticed that Scott was having trouble with his talking, and on one occasion he had said, 'Yes, that was really hard to say.' They were encouraged to continue to be open about the stammer.

Building confidence

Stammering and confidence

The parents of young children who stammer often describe their child as being confident. However, they may have concerns about whether the child's confidence will become undermined by the stammering in the future if it continues. Other parents report that their child lacks confidence, and feel that he would undoubtedly be more confident if he were a fluent speaker. Developing a child's confidence is therefore central to our therapy programme.

Confidence: thoughts and feelings

Confidence is closely linked to the thoughts and feelings we have about ourselves. A child's thoughts and feelings about himself may be affected by what he is being told:

- 'You are so good at helping me to wash the car.'
- 'You are a fast runner.'
- 'You are naughty!'
- 'You are very careful at colouring in.'
- 'You are a very messy girl!'

A child develops a mental vocabulary about himself, based on the feedback he receives. These constructs of 'Good things about me' form the basis of the child's self-confidence.

Giving children feedback

Developing a child's confidence therefore involves influencing what the child thinks and feels about himself. This is more that just a behaviour modification programme, where a child is praised for desirable behaviour. Giving a child positive feedback such as 'well done', 'great', 'good boy' may make the child feel appreciated, and may increase the likelihood of him repeating that behaviour. However, such generic, non-specific words of praise are less likely to help the child generate a positive image of himself. Instead, the child may be given feedback about a specific attribute that has been demonstrated in his actions, such as, 'You put all the toys away, that was very *helpful* of you'. The child will then consider himself to be a helpful person. The feedback the child is given has two components:

- A description of the action which is the focus of praise. This ensures that the feedback is specific, for example, 'You came to get me when your brother fell over and hurt himself...'
- A word or phrase which summarises the child's attribute, for example, '... that was very kind and caring of you.'

This programme of specific, descriptive praise is an adaptation of the model suggested by Faber and Mazlish (1980).

Sincerity

Clearly, it is essential that praise is sincere in order for the child to build up an accurate self-image. If we praise a child for something he has not done, the child might be confused. Moreover, if we over-exaggerate praise, the child may not accept it. Children can be realists with an accurate estimation of how they are performing or what others think of them.

Consistency

Noticing a positive action or attribute in a child may also heighten our awareness that the child is not like that all the time. It can then be tempting to point this out to the child: 'You got into bed without being asked, what a sensible boy! *Why can't you always do that, instead of messing around for ages?*' The warm glow that the child may start to feel, as well as the positive self-image based on how sensible he is, may rapidly dissipate by the end of the sentence. The praise is being given in one breath and taken back in the next.

The language of praise

If a child is to learn and assimilate a positive vocabulary about himself he needs to hear these words frequently. Parents' language needs to be at an appropriate level for the child's comprehension. For a younger child, a more simple vocabulary may be appropriate, for example *helpful*, *kind*, *grown-up*, *careful*, *thoughtful*, *sensible*. As the child develops linguistically, more sophisticated terms can be used, such as *reliable*, *sympathetic*, *loyal*, *conscientious*, *independent*, *observant*.

Reactions to praise

Reactions to praise are interesting. Reacting to praise with a simple 'thank you' shows acceptance and appreciation of the praiser's comments (even if the recipient does not agree with that opinion). Some people are clearly uncomfortable about receiving praise and will dismiss it as if it is undeserved, for example: 'I like your trousers', 'What, these old things? I've had them for ever and couldn't find anything else to put on'. This type of self-effacing reaction may be more likely in adults, who somehow feel that modesty should prevent them from agreeing with and accepting the praise. However, reacting in such a way may leave the praiser feeling disappointed, having his comments dismissed or contradicted. This may deter him from giving any more praise. Children may be less likely to shun the praise, especially if it is accurate and sincere. Moreover, children often react by agreeing with the praise: 'You brushed your own hair – that was very grown up of you', 'I know, I'm very grown up now.'

Helping parents to build up their child's confidence

Most parents praise their children, and some are surprised that praising is a component of a speech and language therapy programme. For the reasons discussed above, we include it for all children and continue with it throughout therapy.

Handout:
Building my child's confidence

Handout

At the end of the third session we give each parent the handout 'Building my child's confidence' (see Appendix XXI). We ask them to read it at home, answer the questions and consider the suggestions, then bring it with them to the next session.

Feedback

At the next session we ask the parents for their views on the handout and anything they agreed or disagreed with. We look at what they have written on the handout.

Discussion

We reiterate the three steps of the praise model, that is:

- Notice something positive
- Describe what you have noticed
- Give the child a word or phrase to add to his list of 'Good things about me'.

We discuss the temptation to give praise and then take it away, as well as the importance of being sincere and setting a good example in accepting praise from others.

Task

We ask the parents to use the praising method at least once each day during the coming week.

Each parent is given a copy of the 'Praise log' (see Appendix XXIII) to record a daily example of when they praised the child, the words they used and how the child reacted. We ask parents to bring the completed 'Praise log' to the next session.

Building confidence:

- *Notice something positive*
- *Describe what you have noticed*
- *Give the child a word or phrase to add to his list of 'Good things about me'*
- *Be sincere*
- *Be consistent*
- *Show him how to accept praise*

At the next session we read the 'Praise log' and ask the parents to comment on their experiences. Sometimes parents of younger children find it difficult to think of a range of words to describe their child's attributes. 'Brainstorming' may be useful in generating new ideas. If parents have found it difficult to praise their child we may practise this during the therapy session. For example, we ask the parents to think of something the child has done recently which they could praise. We then ask them to think of a sentence that would describe it and then we might brainstorm a number of adjectives which they could use, for example:

'When you coloured that man's face you didn't go over the lines. You are a very careful boy.'

'I can see so many colours on the picture now, it looks really lovely. That was very artistic of you'

Parents continue to praise their child and record this in the 'Praise log' on a daily basis throughout the therapy.

> ***Case study*** *Scott, aged three years*
>
> Session 3
>
> *Scott's parents were given the handout 'Building my child's confidence' (see Appendix XXI) to read, complete and think about at home.*
>
> Session 4
>
> *Scott's parents had both read the handout. His father had written that he was already praising Scott quite often but not using the descriptions. He also said he felt a bit guilty as he realised that he often said to Scott, 'Why can't you do that more often?' We reassured him that this is easily done and discussed the implications. Each parent was given a 'Praise log' and asked to record a daily example of when they praised Scott using the specific praise model.*
>
> Session 5
>
> *Both parents had praised Scott on the previous two days. When Scott took his dinner plate over to the sink his mother had said, 'You saved me having to take your plate over. That was very kind of you.' His father had praised him for helping to put the rubbish out, 'You carried all those bags. That was very helpful of you.' They were told they had given positive feedback well, and asked to continue to praise Scott every day and record it on the 'Praise log.'*
>
> Session 6
>
> *Scott's parents had been praising him each day and recording this. They had noticed that while Scott had not previously reacted to praise, on two occasions he had proudly agreed with their comments.*

> ***Case study*** *Khaled, aged five years*
>
> Session 3
>
> *Khaled's mother was given the handout 'Building my child's confidence' (see Appendix XXI) to read, complete and think about at home.*
>
> Session 4
>
> *She had read the handout. She said that she was quite good at praising Khaled by saying, 'Well done' or 'good boy,' but she had never thought about using the description or the label. She said that she had tried it out on him that morning when he put on his shoes ready for school. She had said, 'You put on your shoes without me asking you. Well done.' She was praised for doing this and there was a discussion about why the handout suggested giving the child a label for what has been praised. Khaled's mother said she remembered that*

it was to 'give the child a list of good words about themselves in their brain.' She was asked what labels she could have used at the end of her praise that morning and she suggested 'helpful' or 'grown up.' She was given a 'Praise log' and asked to record a daily example of when she praised Khaled using the specific praise model.

Session 5

Khaled's mother had praised him every day and recorded the praise on the 'Praise log.' She said that she was beginning to run out of labels, so a brainstorm was done to generate a list of suitable words. She was assured she had given positive feedback well, and she was asked to continue to praise Khaled every day and record it on the 'Praise log.'

Session 6

Khaled's mother had been praising him each day and recording this. She commented that he did not respond verbally when he was praised, but he often looked rather pleased with himself.

Turn-taking

'Normal' turn-taking

There is a notion that socially skilled communicators take turns to talk. This implies that one person talks while others are listening, and when they have finished what they want to say, this is somehow signalled and another person takes their turn to talk. However, observation of almost any group of people talking will reveal that interrupting, overlapping, cutting people off and finishing other people's sentences are common characteristics. There appears to be a level at which this is socially tolerated as acceptable and typical, among both children and adults.

Socially-skilled communicators?

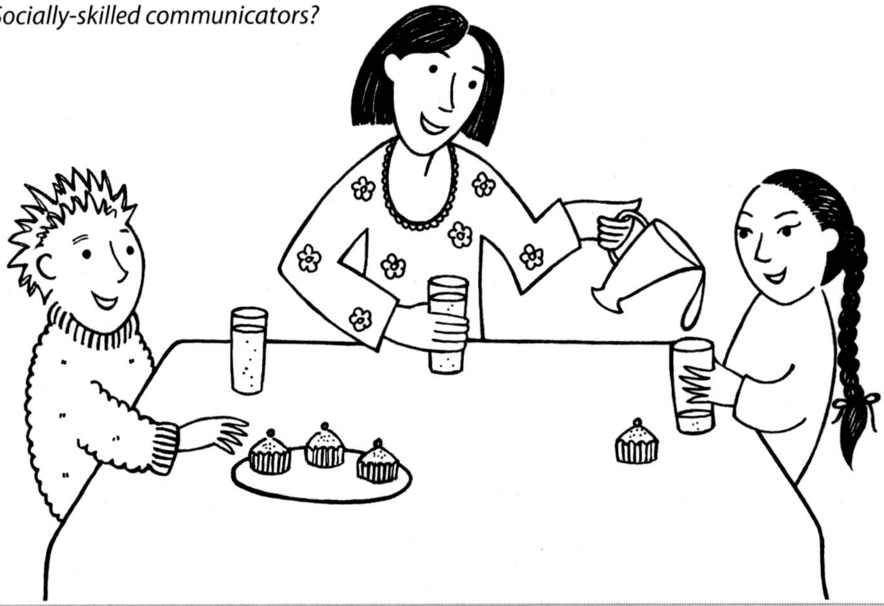

Turn-taking and stammering

Parents sometimes raise the issue of family turn-taking as an area of concern during their assessment.

A number of important issues should be considered regarding children who stammer and turn-taking.

People are sometimes concerned that they should not stop a child who stammers from speaking

Whereas adults might comfortably tell a fluent child to stop talking and let somebody else have a chance to speak, they might be fearful of saying this to a child who stammers. Indeed, many advice sheets have told parents not to interrupt their child or finish his sentences. Instead, the child is allowed to speak for as long as he wishes and others are instructed not to interrupt. There is a risk that the child might develop the habit of speaking at great length, well beyond the limit of his listeners' interest. His fluency may be under greater pressure as he generates more and more language, and he may be in danger of becoming boring.

If a child stammers when he interrupts, he may be more successful at getting a turn

If a child is struggling to talk, his parents may find that they are more likely to allow him to interrupt a conversation. While this is an understandable reaction, it is questionable whether it is fair. The child who stammers is also being given two messages: (1) that interrupting is acceptable, and (2) that stammering when interrupting works very well. The child is not deliberately using his stammer to get a turn, but the stammering is being positively reinforced. An unconscious pattern of behaviour may be being established.

If he is used to being interrupted, the child who stammers may feel he has to speed up in order to finish what he wants to say before he is cut off

This may lead to increased stammering as the child has less time to plan and execute speech fluently.

A child who stammers may not be taking a turn in a conversation

If the child is in an environment with lots of able speakers, he may not have the skills to break into a conversation and others may be reluctant to put him under pressure by inviting him to speak, which may result in him not participating verbally.

Helping parents to improving turn-taking

Handout:
Taking turns to talk

Handout

At the end of the therapy session before the one set aside to discuss turn-taking, we give each parent the handout 'Taking turns to talk' (see Appendix XXIV). We ask them to read it at home, answer the questions and consider the suggestions, then bring it with them to the next session. We also encourage the parents to bring the child's siblings over the age of three to the next session.

Feedback

At the next session, we ask the parents for their views on the handout and look at what they have written. We start with their responses to the observation of the family and we ask the child and any siblings to answer the same questions:

When our family is together:

- *Who does most of the talking?*
- *Who does most of the listening?*
- *Who does most of the interrupting?*

The patterns of turn-taking in the family may be variable: sometimes the child who stammers is dominating turns; in other cases he may not be able to get a word in. Whatever the profile, it is highly likely that the family will benefit from looking at their turn-taking.

Brainstorm

We carry out a brainstorm about why turn-taking is important in a conversation.

Discussion: turn-taking and stammering

We also help the family to consider the relevance of turn-taking to stammering by asking the following questions:

- If the child who stammers anticipates being interrupted, how might this affect his fluency?
- When he interrupts, does it make a difference if he is fluent or stammers?
- What could happen if a child who stammers was never told to stop and let someone else have a turn to talk?

This discussion will help the family understand why turn-taking is important for their child.

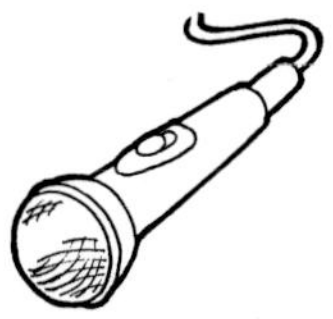

The Microphone Game

We teach the child and other family members the idea of taking turns to talk using the Microphone Game. We explain that we are all going to play a game in the clinic which the family can then play at home.

- We choose an object to be a microphone. This may be a toy microphone or a pencil or a spoon, or any similar object which might represent a microphone.
- We all sit in a circle, with the microphone in the middle on the floor.
- We tell everyone that only the person who has the microphone is allowed to talk and that everyone will have a turn.
- For younger children, the therapist starts by picking up the microphone and saying a word or phrase. Object or verb pictures can be used as a stimulus, or a carrier phrase can be used, for example 'My favourite food is …' When she has finished, she replaces the microphone and somebody else has a turn. This continues until each person has had a few turns.
- Older children are asked to make up a story. The therapist starts by picking up the microphone and starting the story. For example, 'Once upon a time, there was a naughty dog called Bouncer…' The therapist then replaces the microphone and whoever wants to continue the story picks it up. We take turns in a random order rather than in a sequence around the circle.
- The therapist then starts to break the rules, by snatching the microphone from somebody else, by taking a very long turn or by speaking when she is not holding the microphone.
- We ask the family to think of all the rules for the Microphone Game and appropriate turn-taking. We write them down for them to take home. These should include:
  - Only the person who has the microphone is allowed to talk
  - Everybody should get a turn
  - We listen to each other
  - Interrupting is not allowed
  - It should be fair – nobody should have a much longer turn than the others.
- We ask the family to play the game at home, thus further establishing turn-taking in the home environment.
- Another way of doing this is to make a video recording of the family playing the Microphone Game in the clinic, which we then watch to generate the rules as above.

Turn-taking at home

The family plays the Microphone Game at home as often as the parents think it necessary to reinforce the concept of turn-taking. Once the family members are aware of taking turns, the parents often start to remind the family to take turns during everyday speaking situations, for example 'Don't interrupt, Tom has the microphone' (even when there is no actual 'microphone'). One family decided to use a ketchup bottle as a microphone at mealtimes in order to reinforce good turn-taking habits!

> ***Case study*** *Scott, aged three years*
>
> Session 4
>
> *Each parent was given a copy of the 'Taking turns to talk' handout (see Appendix XXIV) to read and complete at home. They agreed that they would bring Scott's sister to the next session.*
>
> Session 5
>
> *Each family member was asked the questions on the handout about the family turn-taking – 'Who does all the talking / listening / interrupting?' Both parents thought that the children talked and interrupted the most and they did all the listening, although Scott's mother said that she often 'switched off.' Scott thought that his sister and his mother talked the most and he interrupted, while his father listened most. His sister thought that Scott talked and interrupted the most and she listened most. There was a brief discussion with Scott's parents about the dynamics between stammering and turn-taking, looking at what was on the handout. The family and the therapist then played the Microphone Game. The family enjoyed this and agreed to play it at home, having decided to use Scott's magic wand as a pretend microphone.*
>
> Session 6
>
> *Scott reported that they had played the Microphone Game twice at home and he wanted to keep playing it because it was fun. His mother said that they had all agreed that she would wave a pretend magic wand to remind them if they did not take turns, and this was working well. She had noticed that both she and Scott's father were joining in family conversations more, and, as a result, the children were taking shorter turns and Scott was much more fluent. It was agreed that the family would continue to play the Microphone Game from time to time, as they saw fit, and continue with the magic wand, real or symbolic.*

Dealing with feelings

Emotions and stammering

'If only I knew what he was thinking or worrying about!'

Parents often report that their child's fluency is affected by his emotional state. They typically find that the child is less fluent if he is frustrated, excited, frightened, anxious or upset, and the child is more fluent when he is feeling calm. Interestingly, 'the jury appears to be out' on the issue of anger – some children become highly fluent when they are angry and others stammer severely.

Whilst all children will experience these various emotions, the depth of feeling and the way the child shows it will vary from one child to another. Similarly, parents will respond to displays of emotion in differing ways: this may be linked to whether they were allowed to express emotion as a child. Culturally, some families do not discuss feelings openly. Parents often tell us that they do not know how to help their child cope with his feelings.

How parents can help a child to cope with how he feels

This model of helping children deal with their feelings is an adaptation of a method suggested by Faber and Mazlish (1980)

Handout:
Helping my child to deal with his feelings

Handout

At the end of the session before the one set aside to discuss the child's feelings, we give each parent the handout 'Helping my child to deal with his feelings' (see Appendix XXV). We ask them to read it at home, answer the questions and consider the suggestions, then bring it with them to the next session.

Feedback

At the next session, we ask the parents for their views on the handout and look at what they have written.

The chart on the first page of the handout helps parents to think about triggers for their child's feelings, how the child shows his feelings and how they typically respond.

Discussion: let it happen

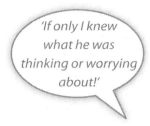

When a child is upset, frustrated or angry it may be a natural reaction for parents to act quickly to try to stop the child feeling as he does. The parent does what he can to make the child feel better, but this may not be showing understanding of the child's emotions. Sometimes it is difficult to accept that a child feels that way. If the parent has noticed that they sometimes respond by telling the child not to feel that way, for example 'Don't be cross', we encourage them instead to allow the child to voice his feelings. This may help the child cope better with his feelings. Waiting while the child cries lets him know that his parent understands that he feels that way, holding him and allowing him to cry, shows concern and acceptance. When a child is frustrated and feeling cross with himself because he cannot do something, his parents might be tempted to tell him it does not matter, he will manage it one day, or they could allow him to vent those feelings and acknowledge his frustration.

Watch and describe

The parents have recorded on the handout (Appendix XXV) how the child shows his feelings. This may be in his posture, facial expression, tone of voice, positioning or actions. The child may be unaware that he is displaying such emotion and he may be unable or unwilling to put it into words. In such cases, we encourage the parents to help him by watching him carefully and describing what they observe, for example:

'I see a very cross face, and those hands are banging on the floor really hard.'

'You look so disappointed about what happened, your face is so sad and your voice sounds very upset.'

By describing what they see, the parents are showing the child that they are aware of his feelings, they are allowing the child to feel that way and they are giving him a vocabulary to verbalise the emotions.

Accept that he feels that way – try not to contradict him

The parents have also recorded their typical responses on the handout. They may have noticed that they sometimes try to help by contradicting the child, for example:

Child: *'I hate the baby.'*
Parent: *'No you don't, how could you say that? She's so sweet and she really adores you.'*

Child: *'I don't want to go to preschool today.'*
Parent: *'Don't be silly, you love it there. You'll be fine once we get there.'*

Child: *'I'm scared of the dark.'*
Parent: *'There's nothing to be scared of. I'm still downstairs and nothing can hurt you.'*

When parents contradict the child, they are telling him that he does not feel that emotion, and hope they are helping the feeling disappear. We encourage parents to believe their child and not to contradict him, in order to encourage him to express his emotions.

Putting the feelings into words

Parents can put the child's feelings into words for him, thus letting him know he has been heard and understood. This might help him to feel less upset and more able to cope with that feeling, for example:

Child: *'I hate the baby.'*
Parent: *'You are finding it really hard to get used to having her around. It makes you feel very cross. Let's think about what we should do in our Special Time together.'*

Child: *'I don't want to go to preschool today.'*
Parent: *'Sometimes you feel upset thinking about going there and you want to stay at home.'*

Child: *'I'm scared of the dark.'*
Parent: *'You're frightened when it's dark and you can't see things so well. Let's think about how we can make it better.'*

Find ways to help him vent his feelings

Some children seem to have a natural tendency to hide their sadness, anger or fear rather than displaying them directly. We may help parents to consider how they can encourage their child to vent his feelings, for example:

- Shouting or screaming as loud and as long as he can (in an appropriate environment!)
- Using a pillow as a punch bag and encouraging the child to pummel it as hard and as long as he can
- Having specially designated scrap paper or an 'Angry Book' that may be scribbled in or torn or 'pictures' drawn of how angry he is
- Set an appropriate example in the way you vent your own feelings
- Say 'It's OK to cry, have a good cry'
- Watch a sad video or read a sad story together to 'unlock' the child's sadness
- Don't be afraid to cry in front of the child sometimes.

It is important to:

- Let the feelings happen
- Watch and describe
- Accept that he feels that way – try not to contradict him

- Put his feelings into words
- Find ways to help him vent his feelings.

Difficulties with separation

Some children separate from their parents with no anxiety and others find it extremely difficult, causing distress to all parties. Being left with a childminder or babysitter may be their first experience of separation, or it may come later when the child starts at preschool or school.

When parents tell us that their child is having difficulties with separation we discuss with them some ideas which might help.

- A routine will often help a child to manage a separation, for example a hug, a kiss and a secret signal which means something special to the child.
- Some children are comforted by keeping something with them which belongs to the parent.
- It may be appropriate to show the child on a clock when the parent will be returning, or describe when they will return, such as after story time, after bath time.
- Some children may fear they are missing out on something exciting while they are separated, so if the parents say they will be doing something which the child does not like, such as going to the supermarket or tidying up the bedroom, this may make the prospect of being apart more attractive.
- In some cases it is the parent who is suffering as much or more than the child about the separation and exploring this with them may identify how to handle it more comfortably.

We may explore with the parents possible reasons for the child's anxiety about separation. It is possible that it is related to a fear that the parent will not return. If the parent is often delayed, this fear is reinforced and the anxiety is unlikely to reduce. We may need to help parents to consider how they can avoid being late to collect their child and have contingencies in place, which the child understands, should they be unavoidably detained. Furthermore, the child may find it easier to cope with his anxieties about separation if he is encouraged to express his feelings, as described above.

Case study *Scott, aged three years*

Session 5

Scott's parents were each given the handout 'Helping my child to deal with his feelings' (Appendix XXV) to read and consider at home.

Session 6

Scott's parents had read the handout and they had both completed the chart on the handout. They had noticed that they often tried to make Scott feel better by telling him not to cry or be cross, and they had both tried to stop themselves from saying this, and instead to just let him feel the way he did.

High standards

High standards and stammering

Some children seem to be born with a natural tendency to always want to get things right. They may also be competitive, never happy with second-best. Being late, colouring over the line, not winning a game, getting something wrong, not being able to do up a button: any of these things can cause great upset or frustration. If the child has exceptionally high standards or is highly competitive he may face difficulties in all sorts of areas, including speaking.

Society often encourages and rewards very high standards in children. Teachers like neatly presented work, careful drawing and attention to detail. Parents appreciate a child who is naturally tidy or who takes care to do a task properly. A competitive spirit is often admired, for example in the sports arena or in academic achievement. So a child who sets himself very high standards is likely to have this reinforced rather than discouraged. As a result he puts himself under greater pressure to get it right, to do better and to be dissatisfied with mistakes or coming second.

High standards
↓
High anxiety
↓
More stammering

Some children who stammer may be aware that their speech is not like other children's, they realise they are making 'mistakes' and they do not like it. If the child is highly sensitive he may be even more aware and upset by episodes of stammering. His distress about his stammering increases his anxiety, which makes him more likely to stammer. If the child can set himself slightly lower standards, he may be less conscious of his speech difficulty. This may then reduce his anxiety about speaking, which may lead to an increase in fluency.

Facilitating a child's fluency may involve helping him to become less sensitised to how he speaks, more tolerant of stumbles and able to accept 'good enough' rather than 'perfect'. Parents may play a key role in helping the child to make these changes.

Helping parents to manage their child who has very high standards

Handout:
The child whose standards are too high

Handout

At the end of the session before the one set aside to discuss high standards, we give each parent the handout 'The child whose standards are too high' (see Appendix XXVI). We ask them to read it at home, answer the questions and consider the suggestions, then bring it with them to the next session.

Feedback

At the next session, we ask the parents what they thought about the handout and look at what they have written.

Discussion: 'a model of imperfection'

Parents aren't perfect

It is highly likely that a child who sets himself high standards will have one or both parents who do the same. This may be nature or nurture, but in either case, the parent is likely to be consciously or unconsciously reinforcing such traits. If the child is to set himself slightly lower standards, the parent may have to model this behaviour first. A parent can help the child to learn that parenthood or adulthood is not about getting it right all the time: life can go wrong, we may lose our job, crash the car, fail an exam, miss a penalty. As children witness their parents managing these events, they will learn to set their own standards, as well as how to react when these are not achieved.

So when a parent comes home from work and says he has had a terrible day, when he got things wrong or he fouled up in some way, he may be helping the child to regard imperfection as acceptable. This can also be done in small ways when parents make a mistake, drop something, lose something or get something wrong. The parent's reaction can set an example of how to handle 'mistakes'. Their natural reaction might be anger, distress, even devastation that something is wrong. But the model of imperfection will react more casually, acknowledging what happened but accepting it as something that happens from time to time.

Modelling reactions to mistakes

To help parents consider how they can present 'a model of imperfection' we ask them the following questions.

'How might your reaction to your own mistakes help your child to lower his unrealistic standards?'

If the child witnesses his parent's distress that the lunch did not turn out well, this is what he will learn. But if the parent shows acceptance and humour at his own shortcomings, the child will see there is an alternative:

'Oh dear. What a silly daddy I am, I forgot to turn the oven on.'
'Oops. Butterfingers. That's the second thing I've dropped this morning.'
'I've lost my keys again. Silly me. I'll have to use the spare ones.'
'Look at me, I've done my buttons up all wrong!'

If the child witnesses his parents making mistakes and reacting in a low-key fashion, his perception of keeping standards may begin to shift. He will also be exposed to alternative ways of reacting when things go wrong for him.

'When your child doesn't get something quite right, how could you react in a way to help him lower his high expectations of himself?'

The parent's reaction to the child's attempts are equally important – focusing on what has gone well rather than what is wrong with it, for example 'You have used so many different colours in this picture, it must have taken you ages to work so hard on it.'

Parents can also help children who set themselves very high standards by thinking about whether they reinforce these tendencies in their responses to the child. Even in the preschool years, competition is rife and society celebrates the winner and ignores or even penalises the loser. Preschool sports days, swimming lessons with badges and certificates, being selected to sing or dance, showing the best paintings or models: there are endless examples of the spirit of competition and 'the best' being rewarded. The school environment may become even more intense, with spelling tests, reading levels, graded tables, house points and national assessments. The child will be receiving messages constantly about how successful or otherwise he is, and a parent can help to reinforce or counter this opinion. For example:

Child: 'I got eight out of ten for my spellings.'

Possible responses:

Parent: 'Well done, you have learned a lot of new words this week.'
Parent: 'What did the other children get?'
Parent: 'Which ones did you get wrong?'
Parent: 'Oh no. You worked so hard on those!'
Parent: 'You're getting better. Perhaps next week you'll get nine.'

Case study *Scott, aged three years*

Session 5

Scott's parents were each given the handout 'The child whose standards are too high' (Appendix XXVI) to read and consider at home.

Session 6

Scott's mother found the handout very interesting as she recognised her own tendency to 'expect a lot of myself and others.' She had tried to be 'a model of imperfection' when she was setting the table, and she said that she thought doing more of this might really help Scott expect a bit less of himself.

Sleep

Many parents report that their child's fluency is worse when he is tired. Ensuring that the child is getting enough sleep therefore seems to be an obvious step in helping him to be more fluent. However, this is an area that parents often find challenging to manage and, if they are seeking help, we often explore the issue with them as part of therapy.

The problems

Many children just do not like going to bed, no matter how tired they are. For a young child, bedtime may signify ending all the fun, missing out on what the rest of the family is doing, being alone, being in the dark, hearing strange noises and having time to worry. Bedtime may occur just at the time that a parent gets home from work, or when visitors have arrived. The bedroom might also signify some kind of punishment, either explicitly, 'that was a very naughty thing to do – go to your bedroom', or, more subtly, when a parent needs some peace and space.

For parents, getting a child off to sleep may have become a great challenge. Various strategies may have been tried along the way – rocking or stroking the child to sleep, having the child in the parents' bed, or the parent sleeping in the child's room. The transition from the parent helping the child to fall asleep to the child getting himself off to sleep can be difficult.

Helping parents with their child's sleeping

Before embarking on a well-intentioned bedtime management programme, we must consider cultural issues, for example if the extended family and social network operates in a different way. In many cultures children are not expected to go to bed in the early evening, especially if there has been a 'siesta' during the day. We therefore find out from parents what they consider to be typical bedtime hours and routines.

Things that may not help a child to go to sleep

We explore with parents what might be preventing the child from getting a good night's sleep.

'But I'm not tired!'

We ask parents to think about whether the child is sufficiently tired when they put him to bed. Many small children need a daytime nap but there may be a transitional period when they still get very tired during the day, but a daytime sleep makes it harder to go to sleep at night. The solution is to prevent the child from sleeping during the day but this is not always easy. Children often fall asleep when travelling in a car or buggy. Parents cannot keep watch over the child all the time to check he has not dozed off. However, parents may find it helpful to restrict the length of their child's daytime sleeping if they are attempting to get them to sleep earlier at night. Sometimes they find that the earlier the nap in the day, the easier it can be for the child to get to sleep at night.

Eating and drinking before bedtime

Parents may need to consider whether the child is having trouble falling asleep because he has just eaten a main meal or if he has had food or drink that contains additives which might stimulate him.

A bedroom full of exciting alternatives

The child's bedroom may be making it difficult for him to go to sleep. Children's bedrooms often house their toys, but they may also have televisions, games consoles, music systems, computers and other exciting pieces of equipment which tempt the child away from trying to go to sleep in bed. Some children habitually fall asleep in front of the television, but what they watch may affect the quality of their sleep.

Exciting activities before bedtime

We ask parents if there is anything that the child typically does at bedtime that might be making it harder for him to go to sleep. A trampoline session on the bed just before bedtime may be a lot of fun and a nice way to end the day with a child, but there is a risk that the child will become 'hyped up' and find it more difficult to relax and go to sleep.

Agreeing and establishing a bedtime

We try to help parents to decide an appropriate bedtime for the child in order to establish a routine. There are no hard and fast rules of exact times that a child should go to bed at a given age, because all children and households are different. Some children need more sleep than others, and most young children sleep for at least 10 hours at night, with the preschoolers also having a daytime nap.

With each birthday, a child's bedtime may become later as a privilege of being older. A younger sibling may resent this, but it can help the older child to feel special and more independent, and the younger child will learn that his bedtime will change as he gets older.

Parents may need to explain to a child why the bedtime is being fixed. They could encourage the child to think of all the benefits of not being tired. Some children may be aware that tiredness affects their speech and they may be more willing to negotiate an earlier bedtime or a bedtime routine if they think it might help their speech.

Helping a child to fall asleep

We discuss with parents the following tips for helping a child to go to sleep.

Routine

Routine seems to help a child, both physically and mentally, to go to sleep. The body develops its own clock, expecting sleep at a certain time and for a certain period. Parents often find that establishing a routine for a child may remove some of the uncertainty, helping the child know what to expect and helping him to automatically comply without the need to challenge. We may explore with parents the kind of routine they could put in place to take the child from the evening mealtime, through bathtime, to going to bed and falling asleep. Some parents prefer a fairly rigid arrangement whereas others have a routine which is looser but nonetheless effective.

Bathtime

We may suggest a warm bath before bedtime to help the child relax and wind down in preparation for sleeping. Bathtimes can also be great fun and parents may need to ensure that excitement does not build through boisterous games.

A drink

A drink at bedtime may be part of the child's routine, signalling that it is time to sleep. We caution parents against drinks with additives which might make it more difficult for the child to sleep, and too much liquid may result in the child's sleep being disrupted by trips to the bathroom.

Bedtime story

We suggest reading a story when the child is in bed to help him unwind in preparation for sleep. Parents may need to consider the content of the book if their child is affected by vivid or frightening storylines.

Managing the separation

A child may be reluctant to be left alone at bedtime. We explore with parents whether comforters, in the form of teddy bears, special blankets, dummies, thumb-sucking and so forth, might help the child. As a child grows older, parents may wish to stop the use of a dummy or thumb-sucking. If the child is going through a period of stammering this may not be the optimal time to try to stop comfort behaviours, so we may ask parents to consider delaying this.

Parents sometimes tell us that they lie down with their child until he goes to sleep. We might discuss the implications of this if it means that the child cannot go to sleep without the parent being there, for instance with a babysitter.

Dealing with fears

Parents often tell us that the child is having trouble sleeping because he is afraid. We help the parents to explore solutions to these fears. Many children are scared of the dark and the use of nightlights or leaving the bedroom door ajar may be useful. They can also be frightened by noises or shadows. Parents can help allay these fears by encouraging the child to voice his concerns and exploring with the child what is making the noise or the shadow. The child may be less fearful when he realises that the knocking is the heating system, rather than a monster.

Methods of settling a crying child to sleep

We describe these methods to parents who are struggling to cope with a child who cries when he is put to bed. The parents can choose the method they prefer and they may find it helpful to tell the child how they are going to manage bedtimes.

- *The gradual method*: the crying child is left alone in his room with the door ajar. When the child cries, the parent waits for at least five minutes before going in. The parent reassures him for a couple of minutes, then leaves him. The parent uses this method on subsequent nights, increasing the time waited before going in by five minutes each night, that is, the first night wait five minutes, the second night wait 10 minutes, the third night wait 15 minutes and so on.
- *The flooding method*: the parent does not go into the child's room, no matter how long he cries. This method can be much more difficult for parents to use as it can be distressing, but it is usually effective and the child may learn to settle himself more quickly than with the gradual method.

Other sleep issues

Parents sometimes raise other difficulties that they have experienced with their child's bedtimes and sleeping.

Letting the child fall asleep downstairs

A child may prefer to fall asleep on the sofa watching television with the rest of the family and then be carried to bed. We explore with parents the issue of the child not developing the habit of getting himself off to sleep.

The night-time visitor

A child may wake during the night and go into his parents' room. He may form a habit of getting into the parents' bed, which can be difficult for the parents to resist as it is the easiest route back to sleep for everyone. We may need to encourage the parents to break this habit by escorting the child back to his own bed. This may cause the parents a few bad nights, but it will be beneficial for all concerned in the long term.

Nightmares and night terrors

A child who has woken from a nightmare often seeks comfort and reassurance before going back to sleep. We may suggest that the parents explore the source of the nightmare as some children are affected deeply by stories and television images or by their experiences. The parents can then help their child by reducing his exposure to potentially frightening experiences.

Night terrors tend to occur earlier in the child's sleep cycle, often before the parents have gone to bed. The child semi-wakes in great distress, often screaming and shaking. He is in a state similar to sleep walking, not being fully awake and unaware of what is happening. We caution parents against waking the child, but suggest they offer comfort and reassurance, and the child usually goes back to sleep, waking the next day with no recollection of what has happened. Night terrors are a relatively common phenomenon in preschool children and tend to be a phase which passes without any form of treatment.

The early riser

Some children seem to be naturally early risers and they may have had sufficient sleep. However, if the child is waking early and as a consequence is getting very tired during the day, his parents may need to help him to go back to sleep or to sleep through until later in the morning. If the morning light is waking the child, we may suggest blackout curtains. Knowing the time may help the child – even a young child may learn to recognise the number seven on a clock, and a digital clock with the minutes covered over may help the child know if it is time to get up. Alternatively, special clocks are available for young children that show the child it is time to get up, for example with a rabbit's ears going up. If the parents report that they cannot get their child to go back to sleep, we might suggest that the child is encouraged to just rest in his bed, play with a toy, look at books or listen to story tapes until it is time to get up.

Reinforcing change

The child's previous bedtime or sleeping regimen may have brought its own rewards, and for some children changing this may need alternative inducement. For example, a child who enjoys climbing into his parents' warm and comforting bed may see little point in stopping this routine.

Reward systems can be very helpful in reinforcing change. We suggest to the parents that they set up a star chart with the child. They tell the child that he will be given a star for every night that he stays in his bed at bedtime, or for staying in his own bed through the night, or for not getting up before seven. Sometimes parents agree with the child that every time he gets five stars he will earn a small treat, such as a trip to the park or an inexpensive toy. However, for some children the stars alone are sufficient reward (see the section on star charts later in this chapter).

Helping a child to change his sleeping habits:

- *Avoid pre-bedtime stimulants or excitement*
- *Create a bedtime routine*
- *Deal with sleep disruptors*
- *Reward target behaviours*

Case study *Khaled, aged five years*

Session 2

There was a discussion about Khaled's tiredness. When she was asked how she thought this was affecting his fluency, Khaled's mother said that when he was tired he tended to 'ramble on' and he stammered more. He was also grumpier with everybody and there was a lot of arguing, especially about going to bed. She also said that Khaled tended to wake before six o'clock in the morning and would disturb his brother. In a discussion about what happened in the early evenings, Khaled's mother said there was no particular pattern, sometimes he would have a bath before tea and sometimes afterwards. He often watched television and there was usually an argument about wanting to watch the next programme. She said that maybe if they had a fairly fixed routine, he might just get used to that and end up going to bed without a fuss. Khaled was asked to help his mother decide on what order they should do things in the evening. He made lots of suggestions and they agreed on a routine that they would try out for that week.

Session 3

When asked how the evening routine and bedtime was going, Khaled's mother said that it had worked very well and he was going to bed each night at seven o'clock without any fuss. However, he was still waking early in the morning so there was a discussion with Khaled about the problem of him waking up too early and being overtired, and also waking his brother up. A star chart was made in the clinic and Khaled agreed that he would stay in his bed, looking at books until his brother woke up, which was usually between 6.30 and 7 o'clock. He was told that he would get a sticker for his chart every morning when he did this. His mother said that when he had five stars he would be able to choose his favourite meal for tea.

Session 4

Khaled's mother reported that he was now going to bed without any fuss. Khaled proudly showed his star chart with stickers on for every day, and he said that he had pizza for tea on Wednesday. His mother said he had been 'as good as gold' about staying in bed in the mornings. She was advised to keep using the star chart and maintain the evening routine.

Sessions 5 and 6

Khaled's mother reported that he was continuing to go to bed without any protest, and staying there in the mornings. She said that she felt it was 'just his normal way of doing things now'. He still loved to get his stickers and choose his meal as a reward.

Behaviour management

Behaviour and stammering

Many parents struggle to manage specific aspects of their child's behaviour, hence the proliferation of television programmes and books aimed at supporting them. We do not think that a child who stammers exhibits more behaviour problems than other children, but the presence of the stammering problem may make it more difficult for the parents to know how best to manage behaviour.

A tantrum in the supermarket, being unwilling to go to bed or 'antisocial behaviour' may present a different challenge for parents who are anxious about their child's struggle to talk, and who know that the stammer becomes worse when the child is upset. They may do all they can to keep the peace, allowing behaviour that is not normally acceptable in order to avoid a confrontation with the child. This may result in a different set of rules being applied for the child who stammers, which can be difficult and perplexing for his siblings. It sometimes leads to boundaries becoming unclear, which may precipitate further behaviour problems. This pattern of managing the child's behaviour with a different or unclear set of standards may not be deliberate or even conscious. It is often just an instinctive response to the problem of stammering, and all the anxiety that surrounds it.

But telling him off might make his stammer worse!

When parents report that they are finding it difficult to manage their child's behaviour, we discuss with them what they are currently doing, as well as alternative ways of coping with the challenge.

Helping parents to manage their child's behaviour

Handout

Handout: *Managing my child's behaviour*

At the end of the session before the one set aside to discuss behaviour, we give each parent the handout 'Managing my child's behaviour' (see Appendix XXVII). We ask them to read it at home, answer the questions and consider the suggestions, then bring it with them to the next session.

Feedback

At the next session, we ask the parents what they thought about the handout and look at what they have written.

Discussion

We explore with the parents what happens when the child does not behave himself: what does the child do, how do the parents react and what is the child's response. Sometimes we ask the parents how they think they would handle the situation if it were another child who was being unco-operative. This might help them find an alternative strategy for managing the child, but they may need reassurance and support to implement this. We also explore the implications of not setting boundaries, or setting different boundaries, for the child who stammers. Some older children who stammer have reported that the stammer can bring occasional benefits, such as a parent or teacher being less strict or bending the rules.

How to encourage a child to co-operate

We use the Faber and Mazlish (1980) model to help parents to manage their child's difficult behaviour, which is described on the handout (Appendix XXVII) and involves the following steps.

Describe the problem

The parent describes to the child what the problem is, or what they see, in a factual way. This removes the accusation and points towards what needs to be done, giving the child the chance to tell himself what to do, for example:

'This floor is covered in toys, there is nowhere to walk.'
'The television is very loud.'
'This toothbrush hasn't been used this morning.'

Give information

This also helps the child work out what to do, for example:

'Toys get broken when they are trodden on.'
'People cannot hear each other when the sound is high.'
'If we don't use our toothbrush our teeth can go bad.'

Say it with a word

A single word can often be more effective than a whole paragraph. The child may switch off from long explanations and lectures, for example:

'toys'
'sound'
'teeth'.

Talk about your feelings

The parent can be honest about how they feel without verbally attacking the child, for example:

'I don't like looking at all this mess.'
'I get fed up with having to shout over the television.'
'I'm worried about your teeth getting holes, because that really hurts.'

Write a note

Sometimes writing it down is more effective than saying it. A child who cannot read may then ask what the note says, for example:

'Danger. Do not enter. Toy hazard.'
'I can't hear you.'
'Please use me' (on toothbrush).

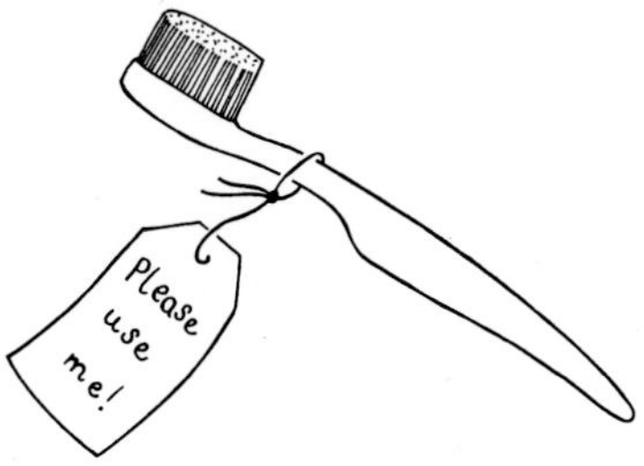

Alternatively, the parent could draw a picture or a sign for the child.

Problem-solving

Parents often tell us that they can feel rather stuck when they are struggling with a problem. They may feel as if they have tried everything and nothing works. We teach the parents how to use problem-solving. This can be helpful as it encourages creative thinking, generates a range of potential solutions and therefore some new options.

Problem-solving may take the form of a simple conversation where the parent describes the problem and then asks the child what he thinks should be done:

'We seem to have a problem here. I am always asking you to tidy up your toys, which you don't want to do, and then I get all cross and it's horrible for both of us. What do you think I should do about it?'

This simple form of problem-solving is particularly useful with a young child.

Alternatively, parents can do a written problem-solving exercise. This may be done with the whole family or just with the child.

The steps are described on the 'Managing my child's behaviour' handout (see Appendix XXVII) and are as follows.

Choose a problem

Someone identifies a problem that they have in everyday life. It has to be the person's own problem, not something that is annoying them about someone else.

For example: the mother wants to solve the problem of always being tired in the morning. She can elaborate why it happens: 'I wake up when XX comes into my bed and then I get hot and it feels so crowded that I toss and turn.' She then writes the problem down, for example:

'My problem is that I can't sleep at night and I am so tired every day.'

Brainstorm a range of solutions

Everyone, including the mother, takes a turn in suggesting a potential solution to the problem and these are written down. In order to encourage creative thinking, no one should react to any suggestion at this stage. The brainstorming process is continued until all the ideas have been noted down.

Evaluate the ideas

The person whose problem it is (in this case the mother) considers each suggestion separately and evaluates the possible impact of each one. She then decides whether to leave it in or take it out.

Rank the ideas

The mother then selects her favourite solution, which she will try first. She also ranks the remaining ideas in order of preference, so that they can be tried if the first idea does not prove to be successful. These ranked solutions are written down.

Try it out!

The mother is encouraged by the others to try out the chosen suggestion and give feedback on what happened.

One of the many strengths of problem-solving is that it encourages children to help their parents to solve a problem, which may be a reversal of the conventional roles. Most people respond positively to being asked to help someone else with a problem; it makes them feel good, their opinion is valued, the other person needs them. Children can be highly imaginative and may help their parents to think 'outside the box'. They may show an unexpected insight into a situation. Sometimes, the mere fact that they are willing to help can change the dynamic of a problem. Children will also learn to develop their own problem-solving skills in this way, rather than the parents always being the ones who provide a solution.

A shift of focus – noticing what is going well

The section on 'Building confidence' earlier in this chapter provides a model of focusing on positive aspects of a child's personality and behaviour, and describing it with a positive label in order to build up the child's confidence. This also gives the child positive feedback for something the parents wish to affirm. It is much easier for all of us to focus on negative behaviours, so that we do not notice what is going well. The structured programme of giving praise and keeping a written log can be very helpful in shifting the focus, which, in some cases, brings about a reduction in the unwanted behaviour.

Setting up 'star charts'

We help parents to develop their use of star charts as a tool to shape a child's behaviour, as described on the handout (see Appendix XXVII).

- We help the parents to set up the star chart in consultation with the child, with an agreed target and reward system.
- We agree with the parents and the child what the target is to be. This should be as specific as possible, such as 'getting dressed on my own'. This will help the child to understand what is required of him and it will help the parents to be clear about what they will positively reinforce. General targets, for example 'being good' are open to interpretation by either party and are not easy to measure or achieve.
- We advise the parents only to set one target at a time in order to make things clear and achievable for the child. Parents may be tempted to add on extra components such as 'getting dressed on my own before breakfast'. Not only is the child expected to get dressed on his own, but he also has to do this before breakfast. This is 'moving the goal posts', and it may become confusing for all concerned if the child fulfils only part of the target.
- We ask the parents to write down the target and draw boxes where the stars will be placed. The days of the week may be included if that is helpful. The parents agree with the child that he will receive a star (or a sticker, a stamp or a tick) when they notice that he has achieved the agreed target.
- When there are two parents, we advise both of them to implement the star chart scheme, although it may need to be agreed who will give the reward to the child.
- We encourage the parents to reward the behaviour as quickly as possible in order to provide immediate and contingent reinforcement. Delayed or inconsistent reinforcement loses its power.

- Some parents decide to offer a 'prize' if a number of stars are won, for example when the child gets five stars they will go to the park. This can obviously increase the child's motivation to change his behaviour to get a star, but we encourage parents to choose low-key tangible rewards. A pet dog or a holiday can be difficult to follow if another star chart is needed in future!
- We encourage the child to bring his star chart to the next session.
- Star charts are usually a short-term method of bringing about a change in behaviour. Once the change has been established, specific reinforcement may no longer be needed, although we sometimes need to remind parents to continue to notice and praise the positive behaviour.

Case study *Khaled, aged five years*

Session 4

Khaled's mother was given a copy of the handout 'Managing my child's behaviour' (Appendix XXVII) to read and complete at home, and to think about the suggestions given.

Session 5

There was a discussion about the issue of managing Khaled's behaviour and his mother was asked to give examples of when she found this difficult. She said that the most difficult aspect of Khaled's behaviour used to be getting him to bed, but now that they had a routine and the star charts, this was no longer a problem. She also said that now he was not so tired, he was a bit easier to manage and there were fewer times when he was awkward. She said that she still found it difficult when they were in the supermarket and he would ask for a toy or sweets. If he was told that he could not have what he wanted he would pester her until she gave in. She said that it was hard because he often stammered when he was agitated about having his own way, and when he stammered she just felt that she had no choice but to give in. There was a discussion about what she had written on the handout about how she would handle this situation if it was her older son who was asking for something. She said that it was much easier to say 'no' to him. The therapist asked what might happen if Khaled realised that he always got what he wanted, if he stammered when he asked for it. It was acknowledged that he might not be doing it on purpose, but a pattern might set in. Khaled's mother decided that she wanted to be firmer with him and when she said 'no' she would not relent, even if he was stammering. She decided that she would try this during the coming week and report back on how it went.

Session 6

Khaled's mother said that they had been to the supermarket three times and on the first occasion he had asked for sweets and she had said 'no'. He protested and she said that she remembered something written in the handout about talking to the child about the problem. She told Khaled that she did not know what to do because he always asked for sweets or toys and she did not have enough money to keep buying them. Khaled said that she should get some more money from the bank, but his mother said there was still not enough, and she didn't know what to do when he kept asking her. He said that he would only ask her if he wanted something really badly. She said that was a good idea and they would try it out. On the next shopping trip, he did not ask for anything, and on the third trip he asked for sweets. His mother told him that they did not have enough money and he replied 'OK Mummy.' Khaled's mother was delighted with this and she was praised for her memory of the handout and her quick thinking in the supermarket. It was agreed that she would continue to try to stand firm when she said 'no,' and she would also ask Khaled to help her next time there was a similar problem.

Routines

Routine and fluency

During the case history we ask parents if their child likes to have a routine. It seems that some children are not particularly bothered about routine, but many parents tell us that their child seems to prefer a routine, for example he likes a particular bedtime sequence. If family life is very busy, some parents find that having a routine in place helps them to be more organised.

Sometimes parents link the fluctuations in their child's fluency to changes in routine, for example the child may stammer more when the family is away on holiday and the usual routines are not in place.

Parents may also tell us that they think it might help the child's fluency if their family had more of a routine. They think that if the child knows what is going to happen, his life will have a level of predictability which might help him to feel calmer and therefore be more fluent.

Helping parents to establish a routine

It is not always easy to establish a routine; households needs to be run with a level of flexibility and this may prevent a regular routine developing. We have often found that, once parents have identified this as an issue for their child, they sort it out without any help. However, if they ask for support, we help them to explore how they can establish a routine at home:

- We discuss the various daily activities and when and how they would like to set up routines

- A morning routine before preschool or school, or a pre-bedtime routine can often offset some of the urgency and tensions that may be arising
- It may be helpful if the parents discuss with the child what the routine should be
- Parents may also need to explain that sometimes things will vary, such as at weekends or on holiday.

Pace of life

Parents often tell us that their family has an extremely busy lifestyle: both parents may be working long hours, 'nine-to-five' having been consigned to history, as evening and weekend working becomes more practical to fit in with child-care and other arrangements. Children may have extra activities: after-school club, play schemes, football, swimming lessons, cubs, brownies or dance. Homework often places extra demands on the parents' and child's time, with reading practice or worksheets to be completed.

Fluency

Although there is no research evidence linking busy households and stammering, many parents tell us that their child's fluency deteriorates when he is in a hurry or rushing to say something, whether it is self-imposed or arising from the situation.

Some children become highly anxious about time-keeping – fearing being late for school or missing the beginning of something. This anxiety and sense of urgency may have a negative effect if the child's fluency is vulnerable to breakdown.

Helping parents to slow the pace

The parents may be using interaction strategies to help their child to take his time (see Chapter 6).

We may help parents to think about their family schedule:

- Writing up the family's weekly timetable can help parents look at the logistics of their arrangements
- They may be able to put in place routines which will help to slow the pace down
- It may be that the responsibilities can be re-assigned, or extra help can be arranged, for example a lift share, in order to slow down the pace

- The various commitments and activities can be discussed, perhaps involving the children, to see if any are no longer appropriate
- Last-minute rushing may sometimes be avoided by a pre-emptive strike – packing the school bag, choosing tomorrow's clothes or making the packed lunch the night before
- The child may be given responsibility for a part of a routine, for example putting his toys away at the end of the day.

Emerging issues

Periods of change and stammering

Many parents have told us that their child's fluency deteriorates during a period of transition or disruption. We can help parents to make sense of this by revisiting the multifactorial model with them. We recall the factors that are likely to have been relevant in the onset of the stammering. We can then look at any new factors which may have come into play as a result of the change in the child's life, to understand how these might be affecting the child's fluency. For example:

- *Physical*: the child may be tired because he is getting less sleep or his day might be more demanding physically
- *Speech and language*: the child might be speaking more in a new environment or he might be using a different language
- *Environmental*: the child might be in a new environment with different routines and greater demands
- *Psychological*: excitement, distress or anxiety may affect the child's speech, especially if he is particularly sensitive.

We identify these factors with parents and then discuss ways of minimising these effects, for example preparing a child for change and encouraging him to express his feelings.

It is often difficult to maintain routines during periods of transition and it is possible that parents may have stopped doing Special Times with the child. We may need to help them to reinstate Special Times, so that there are times when the child is getting his parents' undivided attention and they are focusing on using interaction styles that help their child to be more fluent.

Starting or changing preschool or school

We may suggest that parents try to prepare a child when he is about to start at preschool or school, in order to reduce some of the anxieties and separation issues.

- A visit or series of visits before the child starts may help him to familiarise himself with the geography, staff, children, activities and some of the routines.
- Storybooks about starting at preschool or school are available, and discussions about what to expect may be helpful. Although it is useful to build up a positive image of the new start in the child's mind, it may be unhelpful to make it sound too exciting, otherwise the new experience might turn out to be disappointing for the child, and he might decide at the end of his first day that he has tried it out and does not wish to go back!
- Knowing another child who attends the preschool can often help in settling the child more easily. Arranging 'playdates' prior to starting can facilitate this.
- A child may also benefit from choosing a new bag to take to preschool and deciding what items will be placed inside for the first day such as a lunch box or a favourite toy.

Nurseries and schools will have different policies on how best to settle a child. For some, the parent is expected to stay with the child for a period of time, gradually staying for shorter periods, whereas others expect the parents to leave the child on the first morning and let the staff deal with any separation issues. The nature of the policy may affect the parents' choice of preschool or school, according to their child's temperament.

Holidays

Parents often report that the child's fluency seems to be affected by changes between time at home and away on holiday, or between term time or preschool and school holidays. Whereas we might expect a child to become more fluent during school holidays, when there is no academic pressure and a more relaxed lifestyle, many parents report that their child tends to stammer more when he breaks up from school. This may be because the child's daily life no longer has a pattern, regular bedtimes are abandoned, mealtimes may be more ad hoc affairs and there is little predictability to life.

We sometimes explore with parents how they might build a consistent and predictable routine for their child while they are on holiday, in order to facilitate his fluency, for example thinking about regular mealtimes and helping the child to have enough sleep.

Parents have often found that doing Special Times on holiday helps to maintain the child's fluency.

Parents have told us that it helps the child when they prepare him for the forthcoming changes by talking them through, showing pictures and answering questions. However, building excitement may be counterproductive for fluency!

Moving home

Moving home is reported to be one of life's great stresses, and that is just for the adults! For some children it may be viewed as a great adventure, or it may bring anxiety and a desire for things to remain the same. Moving home might have a further impact if the child's fluency is vulnerable.

We explore with the parents ways in which they can help the child to cope with the change:

- Taking the child to see the new home and talking through the changes might be helpful for the child
- If appropriate, he may choose which room will be his bedroom and plan how he would like to organise his furniture and possessions
- Having photographs of his old house, garden or bedroom might also reassure the child
- Encouraging the child to show his feelings about moving may help him to cope better.

Separation and divorce

A breakdown in the parents' relationship is likely to affect a child's life in both practical and emotional terms, which may also affect his fluency. There may be tensions and discord in the home as the relationship deteriorates, followed by the disruption of separating into two homes, allocating resources and working out the arrangements for custody and access.

We may help the parents to find a source of support as they go through this process, which may reduce the impact on the child. It can be difficult for a parent who is in distress to help their child to cope with the complexities of this situation.

If a parent tells us that they feel too upset to cope with the child's feelings as well as their own, we might suggest that they find someone for the child to talk to, for example a family friend, a teacher or us as their SLT.

We may need to help parents understand how difficult it might be for the child if he is encouraged to take sides. The breakdown of the parents' relationship with one another need not necessarily undermine the relationship that each parent has with the child, and maintaining this relationship will help the child to cope with all the changes.

It would be very natural for the child to be stammering more and we explain to the family that this is to be expected. We can also reassure them that the stammering is likely to improve once life has settled down.

We can recommend resources to help the child and family through this time (see the Resources section later on).

Bereavement

Helping a child to cope with loss can be difficult, especially if the parents are suffering with their own feelings of grief. The subject of death carries certain taboos and parents may think it necessary to protect the child from the harsh realities of loss. A child's first experience of loss may come with the death of a pet, when parents can help children to learn to understand death and the feelings associated with it. If the loss is of a family member or a friend we may help the family access support.

We can explore with the parents how they might help their child to cope with loss:

- Some children find it easier to cope if they are better informed about what happened and what the future holds. We can suggest that the parents encourage the child to ask questions, showing that they are prepared to talk about what is happening.
- Parents may help by allowing the child to show or verbalise his emotions, answering questions and sharing their own feelings.
- We recommend books or videos to help children who are suffering a loss, for example *Bambi*, *Dumbo* or *Finding Nemo*. These may encourage the child to talk about how he is feeling, or just cry.

Conclusion

In this chapter we have outlined a range of family strategies that can be used with families of children who stammer. We have found that when they are implemented in conjunction with the interaction strategies described in Chapter 6, many of the children need no further treatment, only review and monitoring. However, if the child's fluency continues to be a cause for concern, in Chapter 8 we describe child strategies which may be useful as a further stage in the therapy programme.

8

Child Strategies

To recapitulate, Palin Parent–Child Interaction therapy (Palin PCI) aims to facilitate a child's fluency by developing his skills in the context of a supportive environment. We include interaction strategies so that parents will develop the interaction styles that help the child to be more fluent, as well building up his underlying speech and language abilities. We use family strategies to develop the child's confidence, his ability to cope with his feelings or any other relevant behaviour management or helpful family routines. Our research has shown that most children achieve fluency with the interaction and family strategies (see Chapter 1). However, some children's fluency continues to be a cause for concern and we introduce direct fluency therapy at this stage. We expect parents to continue to do Special Times and their targets with the child, as well as implementing other family strategies.

The child strategies teach the child what he can do to help himself. The interaction and family strategies have created an environment in which the child is more likely to be able to use these child strategies.

> **Child strategies:**
> - *Rate reduction*
> - *Pausing to think*
> - *Easy onset*
> - *Being more concise*
> - *Eye contact/ focus of attention*

Parents remain closely involved in the therapy process. We continue to include both parents if they are available, but are happy to work with just one parent if it is more convenient. Parents observe the activities and we then involve them in a practice activity in the clinic which we ask them to practise with the child at home. This is initially done in addition to Special Times, but once the child is able to generalise the direct therapy strategy into their conversation, it can be incorporated into the interaction within the Special Times.

The speech modification strategies are 'Tortoise Talking', 'Bus Talking' or 'Aeroplane Talking'. Each of these approaches follows a similar format, as follows:

- Introduce the concept
- Introduce the characters in a story

- Identification activity
- Production of strategy at single-word level
- Increase length of sentence
- Generalisation and reinforcement.

Rate reduction: Tortoise Talking

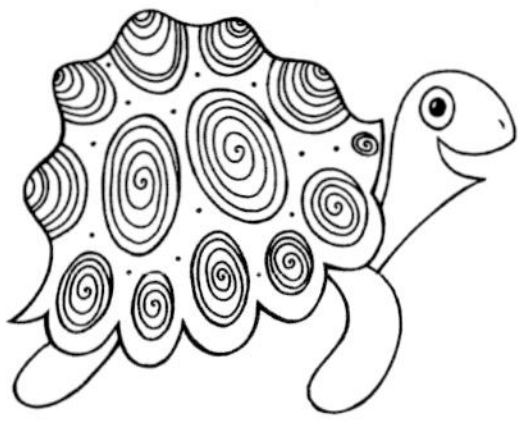

Some children have a natural tendency to speak very quickly, even when those around them are modelling a slow rate, using appropriate pausing and giving themselves time to think and plan what they want to say. This tendency to a rapid speaking rate may be contributing to the breakdown in fluency.

Tortoise Talking is used as a simple method of reducing a child's rate of speech. It is based on Meyers and Woodford (1992) *The Fluency Development System for Young Children*, which teaches cognitively based fluency exercises. The child first learns the concept of speed and then relates this to the act of talking. The parents observe and then join in with the activities as described below.

Teach the concept of fast versus slow

If the child does not understand the meaning of 'fast' and 'slow', we start by teaching the concept, using a variety of toys and games. We play with cars, trains, animals or other characters and categorise them according to their speed.

Once the child understands the concept and its labels, we introduce the characters of the tortoise and the racehorse. We do this by telling the child a story based on Aesop's fable, 'The Tortoise and the Hare' and act out the story with a toy tortoise and horse:

Once there was a racehorse who thought he was the best and fastest animal in the world. He loved to boast about how fast he was, especially to the animals who were not as fast as him. One day he met a tortoise and said to him 'I am the fastest animal in the whole world. I can go faster than anything else, especially you! You are just a slow old tortoise! Let's have a race and I'll show everyone how fast I am'. The tortoise agreed and they lined up. Ready, steady, go! The racehorse gets off to a flying start while the tortoise plods on slowly. The racehorse goes faster and faster until his legs get all tangled up and he falls down. The tortoise just keeps on going at his own slow pace until the finish and, hooray, he wins the race!

Guess who is speaking

We then demonstrate the racehorse speaking quickly and the tortoise speaking slowly, by playing a game where we pretend to be either the racehorse or the tortoise, and the child has to guess who is speaking. For example, looking at pictures of food, we say, 'I like potatoes', using an obviously fast or slow rate and the child guesses which animal is talking. After the child has correctly guessed several times, we ask, 'How did you know that it was the racehorse?', thus encouraging the child to use the labels 'fast' and 'slow' in relation to speech.

Role reversal

We then swap roles, and the child pretends to be either the tortoise or the racehorse and the therapist does the guessing. The child has therefore learnt to discriminate between the two rates of speech and is now producing the contrast.

Involve the parent in the session and at home

Once the child is competently contrasting the fast and slow rate, we involve the parent in the activity, taking the role of speaker or listener. We then ask them to play the game at home.

Tortoise Talking

When we are satisfied that the child is able to discriminate between fast and slow rates of speech, we focus on production of the slow rate, that is, Tortoise Talking. We start at a single-word level and gradually increase the length and complexity of the sentences, at a pace and level where the child can maintain the slow rate and remain fluent. We have typically found that when a child reduces his rate he speaks fluently. If he does stammer, we ask him to speak even more slowly. If the child has difficulties with onset, and he tends to block, we may have to work on easy onset, using Aeroplane Talking (see below). It is important to ensure that the child can maintain fluency at a particular language level before increasing the length and complexity. Suggestions for activities are given later on in this section.

Handout:
Practice chart

Home practice

Home practice is essential to transfer Tortoise Talking beyond the therapy room. We discuss with the parents the level of the activities so that the child can easily use the slow rate and be fluent. We give the child a practice chart (see Appendix XXVIII), which they can write on or put stamps or stickers on to record what they have done at home.

Tortoise Talking in free play or general conversation

Once the child is able to maintain Tortoise Talking at a sentence level, we introduce it during a free play session in the clinic, with both the parent and the child using it. We then ask them to have Tortoise Talking times at home. It can be fun to suggest to the child that he should monitor his parent's rate of speech and if he hears his parent talking like a racehorse he should remind the parent that they are supposed to be doing Tortoise Talking!

Don't say 'Use your Tortoise Talking'! Praise your child when he uses it

We discourage parents from prompting their child to use Tortoise Talking when they hear the child stammering, as this may result in the child viewing it negatively. Instead, we give parents a chart which they use when they have noticed their child spontaneously using Tortoise Talking. The child is given a sticker or a tick on the chart as reinforcement (see Appendix XXVIII).

Pausing to think: Bus Talking

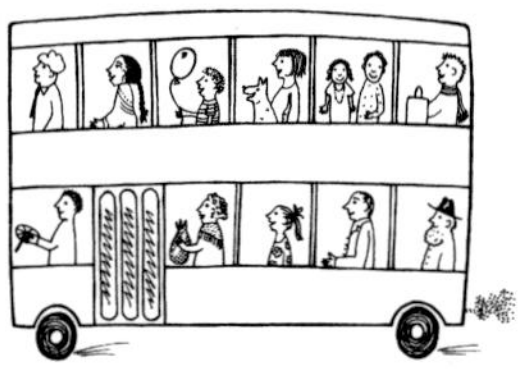

Sometimes a child does not give himself enough time to think and formulate what he wants to say, especially if he has language-formulation difficulties or a word-finding problem. Parents often tell us that their child has a tendency to start to speak before he has decided what he wants to say, and the child may need to develop specific strategies to pause and think in order to build his fluency.

Bus Talking is a development of Tortoise Talking, with the added component of stopping to think before and during an utterance.

Teach the concept of fast versus slow

We introduce the concept of slow versus fast in a similar way to Tortoise Talking, except that the characters are a bus and a racing car. We use a toy bus and racing car, or we build them using Lego® or Duplo®. We play out the story of the race between a bus and a racing car on a circuit (which may be made using Duplo® or a wooden track), with the racing car spinning off on a bend because it is going too fast, and the bus proceeding at a sedate speed to win the race. The bus cannot go fast because it must take care of its passengers and it has to stop now and then to let people off and on.

Guess who is speaking

We then pretend to be the bus, talking slowly with pauses before and between utterances, or the racing car, talking fast with no pauses. The child identifies which one is speaking, and then the roles are reversed. The parents observe, then practise this with the child in the clinic and do further practices at home.

Producing Bus Talking at single-word level

We introduce the production of Bus Talking at the single-word level. Lego® or Duplo® is very helpful at this stage and we build a bus which can accommodate passengers (Lego® or Duplo® people), and a person can be used for each word that the child says.

- We set up the road circuit with two bus stops.
- At each bus stop there are a number of people and a corresponding number of pictures of objects.
- The child slowly moves the bus to the first bus stop, stops to let one person on the bus, then slowly moves away. As the bus moves, the child slowly names the object on the picture.
- When the bus gets to the next stop, it lets the person off the bus, before the next person gets on and the bus 'names' the picture as it slowly moves along.
- This continues until the child has established the pattern of stopping at a bus stop, thinking of the word, then saying the word slowly.

The parents observe and then join in with this activity.

Handout:
Practice chart

Home practice

We ask the parents to practise with the child at home at the single-word level and we give them a practice chart (see Appendix XXIX) as reinforcement. Parents and children often enjoy making a roadway at home with bus stops and a Lego® bus with people.

Bus Talking and increasing sentence length

When the child is able to use Bus Talking at a single-word level, we increase the length and complexity of the sentence, with pausing as an integral feature of each utterance.

We use the roadway with bus stops, people and a bus to help the child move from a single-word level to a sentence level, using slow rate and pausing.

- The bus, with people on board, arrives at a bus stop where there is a picture and two people waiting.
- The child takes the other passengers off the bus before putting the two people on the bus as he thinks of the two words he will say about the picture, for example 'yellow cup'.
- Then the bus slowly moves away and the child says the two words slowly.
- We increase this level as the child becomes accustomed to using Bus Talking. Ultimately, there might be many people at a bus stop and the child always takes the other passengers off first, then puts the people on as he thinks of what he will say before the bus starts moving slowly. With longer utterances, we use lots of pauses.

The parents join in the activity in the clinic and then practise at home at a word level that is easy for the child.

Bus Talking activities

Once the child is able to use Bus Talking at a sentence level, we incorporate it into activities without using the bus going around the roadway, but we may keep the bus on view as a reminder to use Bus Talking. We encourage the child to check that we are using Bus Talking, and not talking like a racing car. We involve parents and suggest suitable activities at home when both the child and the parents will use Bus Talking. Again, children often enjoy being given the role of monitoring whether their parents are using Bus Talking, or whether they are being racing cars. These home Bus Talking practices can be recorded on the practice chart.

When the child is able to use Bus Talking at a sentence level, we incorporate it into practices using free play. The ultimate aim is for spontaneous use of Bus Talking.

Generalisation and reinforcement

As with Tortoise Talking, we discourage parents from prompting their child to use Bus Talking when they hear the child stammering, as this may result in the child viewing it negatively. Instead we give parents a chart which they use when they have noticed their child spontaneously using Bus Talking. The child is given a sticker or a tick on the chart as reinforcement (see Appendix XXIX).

Case study *Khaled, aged five years*

At the end of Palin PCI, Khaled's stammering had reduced, but his rate of speech was still rapid and his mother remained concerned about this and his speech sound difficulties. Bus Talking was introduced because it would help Khaled to give himself more time to plan and execute speech, thus helping his fluency and his phonology. A block of six one-hour, once-weekly sessions was arranged.

Session 1

Khaled and his mother enjoyed acting out the story with the toys and he was able to discriminate reliably between the slow with pauses rate and the fast rate and produce it at a single-word level. They were asked to practise this at home.

Session 2

They had played the guessing game at home and Khaled's mother said that he was very good at hearing and producing the difference between the bus and the racing car. Bus Talking was practised at a two-word level then increased to a three-word level, using the Lego® bus on the road, and the people at the bus stops. Khaled quickly grasped the concept of pausing and then speaking slowly as the bus moved along. His mother joined in and agreed she would continue with this activity at home. She was reminded not to prompt him to use his Bus Talking outside of focused practice sessions.

Session 3

Khaled's mother said that they had been doing Bus Talking with his storybook. They turned the page, then 'waited to let the people on the bus' before slowly describing what they saw. She said that Khaled's speech was 'lovely and slow' when he did this and she thought it even sounded a bit clearer. Activities were introduced at a sentence level during the session and Khaled maintained the Bus Talking consistently. The therapist then explained to Khaled that everybody was going to use Bus Talking while they played with some toys. He was told to listen carefully to his mother and the therapist and if he heard any racing cars, he should tell them to do their Bus Talking. He maintained his Bus Talking very well in free play. Khaled and his mother agreed to practise Bus Talking at home as often as they could, and Khaled was given a chart and some stickers to show the number of times they had practised.

Session 4

Khaled's mother said that he was using his Bus Talking well during the practices, and she had noticed him doing it at other times. He was very proud of the number of stickers on his chart. She said that she thought he was talking more slowly and clearly now. She agreed that she would comment when she heard him using it spontaneously, for example 'That was lovely Bus Talking.' She was reminded that Khaled was still not ready for her to prompt him to use his Bus Talking outside of the practice sessions.

It was decided that it was not necessary to have two further clinic sessions as they had done so well with the Bus Talking. An appointment was arranged for six weeks later and Khaled's mother agreed to practise the Bus Talking within the Special Times.

Review session

Khaled's mother said that he was using Bus Talking consistently, except when he was excited or in competition with other children to speak. She said that other people seemed to find it easier to understand what he was saying, but some of his speech sounds were still not right.

We did a screening of Khaled's phonology and agreed with his mother that we would arrange some therapy sessions to work on his speech sounds (see Chapter 9).

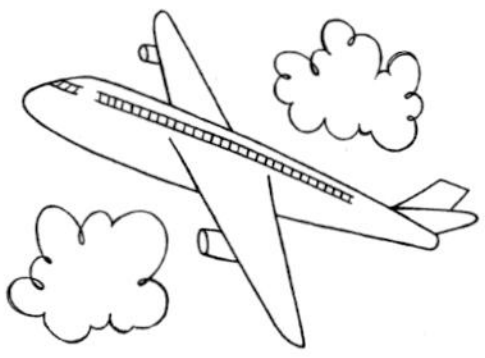

Easy onset: Aeroplane Talking

We have found that rate reduction is usually sufficient to help a child be fluent, but sometimes if he is blocking or struggling with the onset of speech, he may benefit from specific strategies to soften any hard attack or use a gradual onset to speech.

- We introduce the child to the concept of hard talking versus easy talking using Aeroplane Talking: the aeroplane takes off from the ground, gradually getting higher in the sky. We show that the aeroplane does not go from the ground to the sky in a sudden movement, it slowly gains height.
- We do a listening activity with the child when he tells us when he hears Aeroplane Talking: we contrast hard onset ('Was that like an aeroplane?' No) with easy onset ('Was that like an aeroplane?' Yes!).
- We reverse roles so that the child is producing the hard onset versus the easy onset.
- We introduce activities at a single-word level and encourage the child to use Aeroplane Talking.
- We build up the length of the child's sentences using Aeroplane Talking. Many children only need to use easy onset at the beginning of a sentence, not at the beginning of every word.
- The parents observe these activities, then join in and practise them at home with the child at a level which is appropriate for the child.
- We encourage the parents to notice and reinforce when the child spontaneously uses Aeroplane Talking, rather than reminding the child to do so.

Being more concise

Some children find it difficult to express themselves concisely: they tend to talk at length, sometimes losing the point of what they are trying to say, and often with increased stammering. Sometimes these children have specific language difficulties which make it more difficult for them to express themselves concisely. Alternatively, they may have highly sophisticated language skills and they enjoy and are encouraged to talk at length. Parents often describe their child as being 'talkative' and admit that they sometimes 'switch off' and pretend to listen, rather than asking the child to be more concise.

Turn-taking

This is a useful starting point to help a child to be more succinct. If the child who stammers is being allowed to monopolise the family conversations and take lengthy turns, with others feeling wary of interrupting or cutting him short, he will not learn to express himself concisely. See Chapter 7 for turn-taking management.

Being concise

We sometimes have to help the child to reduce the length of his utterances. This may require some metalinguistic ability and we develop this by saying both long and short sentences and asking the child to identify whether they are long or short. With an older child we may count the words and decide together if the sentence is long or short. We can then reverse roles so that the child is producing the contrast between long and short sentences.

Using a composite picture, we ask the child to deliberately produce a long description with lots of words, for example 'The boy is in his bedroom and there are cars and books and a ball and lots of other toys on the floor'.

We then ask him to describe the same picture using fewer words, for example 'The boy's bedroom is messy with toys on the floor'.

When the child is able to reduce the length of his sentences describing pictures, we use conversation tasks, for example 'How did you get here today?'

- *Long*: 'I walked out of my house and got into mummy's car and we drove to the station then we waited for a train then it came and we arrived at the station so we got off then we got a bus and then we walked the rest of the way here.'
- *Short*: 'I came by car, then train, then bus, and then we walked the last bit.'

We then use other verbal activities, for example build a story or sequencing pictures, to help the child practise being more concise, and the parents replicate these activities with the child at home.

Once the child is able to moderate his sentence length in this way, we encourage him to use this skill in his conversation. We ask the parents to notice when he is being concise and reinforce this with some praise, for example 'You managed to explain that very well in a short sentence'.

Talking more succinctly may involve more planning time, so the child might need to use more pausing before he starts to speak in order to produce a shorter utterance.

Secret signal

Some children benefit from reminders to be concise, so we may get the child to negotiate with his parent a secret signal, for example a hand signal. This is for the parents to use when they want to remind the child to keep it short.

Eye contact or focus of attention

Avoiding eye contact is a common feature of stammering behaviour in older children and adults, but younger children are less likely to be looking away deliberately. It is more likely that a young child will have reduced eye contact because he is distracted by other stimuli. If the child is trying to focus on other things while he is talking, it is possible that he is putting himself under too much pressure, which may result in fluency breakdown. He may need to focus visually in order to 'harness' his thoughts, and improving eye contact may be a strategy which achieves this and thereby helps fluency.

We may need to start by helping the child and parents understand that using eye contact does not involve unblinking staring. A speaker often looks away as he thinks about what he is going to say, then looks at his listener when he starts to speak, then looks away when he pauses. The listener tends to maintain eye contact throughout. However, there are cultural differences: for example in some African cultures it is considered insolent to look another person in the eye. We need to be sensitive to these differences and we ask the families or interpreters if we are not sure.

Strategies (see 'Eye contact and talking' handout Appendix XVIII):

- We use role-play to explore how looking and speaking go together. We start by talking to the child but not looking at him, and then we talk and stare, so that the child can identify why looking is important and when it is appropriate.
- We use verbal activities, for example the 'Guess who?' game, Pelmanism, picture lotto, to practise using eye contact.
- The child can choose a secret signal that his parents will use to remind him to look, for example a cough, clicking fingers.
- We ask the parents to reinforce the child's use of eye contact by praising him, for example 'That was really lovely looking'.

If the child is too young for these activities, we help parents to use indirect strategies to gain and maintain their child's eye contact and attention, for example:

- Ensuring that they are at the child's level and in his line of vision
- Ensuring that they are using eye contact with the child
- Waiting until the child is looking at them before saying something
- Using touch, humour or surprise

- Saying the child's name
- Holding the picture or object of attention at the level of their face so that the child is encouraged to look at the parent.

Summary

The child strategies provide the child with techniques which will increase the likelihood of fluency. The various strategies are different, but we use similar methods when teaching and transferring them.

Troubleshooting

What if the parents have the expectation that the child will be able to use the strategy all the time?

When parents hear their child using a strategy and being fluent, it is natural for them to want the child to use that strategy as much as possible. In order to demonstrate to parents how difficult this would be for the child, we sometimes ask the parents to use the same strategy during their conversation with us in the clinic. After about 10 minutes we ask them how they felt they managed and what it was like for them to concentrate on changing the way they spoke, whilst having a conversation. We have typically found that parents quickly realise how difficult it would be for their child to maintain the strategy for any length of time. We remind parents that the child will need to practise using the strategy in focused practice sessions in order to develop this skill to a level where he can use it in everyday conversations.

What if the child manages to use the strategy well in the clinic or in structured activities at home but generalisation is not happening?

We have found that generalisation may be facilitated with the use of star charts. We make the chart in the clinic and tell the child that his parents will be listening very carefully for when he uses his Bus Talking (or whichever strategy). When they hear him using it they will put a sticker on the chart. Initially, the child may need his parents to remind him that they will be listening for when he uses his strategy, for example, during a mealtime, whilst walking to school, or when he talks to grandma on the phone. We ask the child to bring the chart back to the next session to show us how many stickers he has been given.

What if the child becomes very aware of his speech and anxious about it?

If the child becomes aware of his speech and anxious about it in response to direct therapy sessions, we initially check with parents how they are getting on with the practice at home and make sure they are only focusing on his Tortoise Talking (or whichever strategy) during practice time. As described above, when parents hear their child using a strategy and being fluent it is natural for them to want the child to use that strategy as much as possible. They may therefore be prompting the child to use his Tortoise Talking outside of practice time. We remind parents that to begin with we only expect the child to use his Tortoise Talking during focused practice sessions. Only when the child has mastered this do we encourage parents to praise the child when they notice him using his Tortoise Talking spontaneously outside of the practice sessions. Following this stage, some children are happy to be prompted to use their strategy, but we only set this up in agreement with the child, and parents are asked to limit their prompting to a few times each day. We also check with parents how many practice sessions are carried out during the week, when the practice sessions take place and the level of the activities being worked on. We want to ensure that practice sessions are fun and enjoyable for the child, with a focus on success.

What if the child's attention span is not long enough to do the activities?

If a child's attention span is not sufficient to sit and do the activities during the session, we may need to review our decision to work directly with the child. It may be more appropriate to focus on further developing the child's attention skills before working with him directly on his stammer.

What if the parents take a 'back seat' in therapy as they think the focus is now on the child and they do not feel so involved?

Parents continue to be a key component of the therapy even when we are working directly with the child. We actively include parents in the direct therapy sessions right from the start so that they feel involved and understand their ongoing role in supporting their child's fluency. During the session, we demonstrate and model to parents the techniques and activities and then observe the parent carrying out the activity in preparation for doing it with the child at home.

If only one parent is attending the direct therapy sessions, we periodically invite the other parent to a session. We want to ensure that the other parent is kept up to date with the therapy and we identify how they can continue to support the child's fluency at home even when they are not attending on a weekly basis.

Suggestions for activities

- Posting pictures
- Picture dominoes
- Picture lotto
- Pelmanism
- Things that go together
- Kim's game
- Spot the difference
- What's wrong?
- Guess who?

9

Other Strategies

Language or phonology therapy for the child who stammers

In some cases, the child who stammers will also present with a language or phonological problem, or both, that will warrant attention. Therapists often express concern about how to manage these children. They fear that focusing on developing language or speech sound skills may make the child's stammer worse. Indeed, we have seen a number of children who initially presented at a speech and language therapy clinic with delayed speech or language development, and have undergone a period of therapy after which, to the dismay of the therapist and the family, their fluency has deteriorated and they have started to stammer.

> **Other strategies:**
> - *Language or phonology therapy*
> - *School or preschool liaison*
> - *Onward referral*

We recommend therapy to develop the speech and language skills of children who stammer with a language or phonological problem, or both, as their difficulties with language or speech may be:

- Affecting their ability to be fluent
- More of a concern to parents or the child, or both, than his stammer
- Affecting the child's academic progress
- Making it harder for the child to communicate effectively.

Clinical texts on how to treat the child who stammers with a language or phonological problem vary in their recommendations (Bernstein Ratner, 1995; Conture, 2001; Conture *et al*, 1993; Louko, 1995; Nippold, 2004; Wolk, 1998). The various options suggested in these texts include:

- Working on both problems at the same time
- Treating them one after the other
- Treating only one problem in the hope that the other will recover naturally.

There are also differing views on whether treatment should involve indirect or direct methods (see Nippold, 2004).

For children with a language or phonology problem, or both, we typically recommend the indirect component of Palin PCI (interaction and family strategies) as the first course of intervention, while simultaneously monitoring the development of the child's language or phonological skills. The early form of Palin PCI was adapted for use with children with delayed language (Kelman & Schneider, 1994) and is widely used in Early Years settings (Cummins & Hulme, 1997) in the UK. In addition, there are a number of similarities between aspects of Palin PCI and other parent-focused interventions for children with language impairment (Girolametto *et al*, 1986; Manolson, 1992; Weistuch *et al*, 1991). The interaction strategies within Palin PCI will promote the child's overall language and speech sound production skills, as will other family strategies such as turn-taking, without placing extra demands on the child's fluency. Furthermore, strategies which slow the pace of interaction and increase pausing will help the child's speech, language and fluency, as he gives himself more time to think, plan and execute what he wants to say.

Once the Palin PCI programme is completed and the child's progress has been monitored, we would then consider direct therapy for language or speech, or both, as required. If the language or phonological problem is mild and is not affecting the child's effectiveness to communicate, we may wait until the child has made progress in his fluency, and this has been maintained for approximately three months, before beginning a further course of therapy.

Some things to consider when working directly on the language or phonological skills of a child who stammers

Focus on input rather than output skills

We use the usual methods to work on language or phonology, but initially we place more of an emphasis on inputting new skills and concepts, without demanding an increased output from the child. If phonology is the concern, we focus on modelling the sounds to be worked on and develop the child's auditory awareness and metalinguistic skills. We take a tentative approach to correction of the child's speech sound errors as he may become self-conscious about his 'mistakes', and focus more on saying things correctly, which in turn may affect his fluency. We therefore advise parents that if a child makes a speech sound error at home, they can repeat what the child has said, giving the correct model, without asking the child to try to produce the correct form of the word.

Monitor fluency skills

We need to monitor the child's fluency closely whilst working with him directly on his language or speech. We want to maintain a balance between building foundation skills for fluency and increasing demands on the child's system, in order to avoid fluency breakdown. We have found that a period of therapy focusing on speech or language sometimes results in an increase in stammering for a short period of time as the child makes progress in his development. However, we may also need to consider that an increase in stammering may be an indication that too much focus is being placed on the child's speech or language production skills.

Child's speech and language level

When working with the child directly on his stammering (child strategies), we only practise fluency with language and phonological structures that the child has already mastered. We would not expect a child to work on both fluency and language, or fluency and phonology, within the same activity, until we are sure that he is able to make use of what he has learnt at a simple level first.

Case study *Khaled, aged five years*

Khaled attended a course of Palin PCI with his mother, which included four sessions of direct fluency therapy when he learnt to use Bus Talking. His phonological difficulties were beginning to resolve, but there were intelligibility problems that were causing his mother concern.

He attended for six sessions of phonological therapy. Although a focus was placed on practising specific sounds in isolation and in single words, the main focus was on developing Khaled's auditory awareness, specifically targeting his ability to perceive the phonological contrasts. When practising at the single-word level Khaled was encouraged to use his Bus Talking. Home practice also mainly focused on developing his auditory discrimination skills. Khaled's mother was reminded not to correct him, but to provide a model of the word and to praise Khaled when she heard a correct pronunciation. Khaled's production of the phonological contrasts began to develop, despite not being the main focus of the therapy, and his intelligibility began to improve. His progress was then reviewed at three-monthly intervals and he was discharged after one year.

Treating CWS with specific language impairment, attention deficit hyperactivity disorder or an autistic spectrum disorder

Increasingly, we are seeing children who stammer who also have a diagnosis of specific language impairment (SLI), attention deficit hyperactivity disorder (ADHD) or an autistic spectrum disorder (ASD). Little is known about the specific characteristics of stammering in these children, and limited information is available on how to treat children who stammer with SLI, ADHD or ASD (see Healey & Reid, 2003; Healey *et al*, 2005). If a child is referred with an additional diagnosis we recommend a full assessment to gain further information about the child's strengths and vulnerabilities. If a specialist SLT is available within the service, we would also liaise with her to gain further information about the child and the disorder in question. However, a careful analysis of the child's needs will determine whether therapy should focus on developing the child's fluency or on other aspects of his development.

Typically the *indirect* component of Palin PCI is recommended as the initial form of intervention. If we decide to work with the child *directly* (child strategies) to manage his stammering we would make use of guidelines already developed and found to be effective in improving the performance of children with SLI, ADHD and ASD. We would also work closely with the SLT working with the child in preschool or school (if appropriate) and liaise with preschool and school staff.

Summary

In order to understand the nature of the child's stammering and the impact of any coexisting problems we need to carry out a full assessment to understand each child's individual strengths and vulnerabilities. This will enable us to develop an individualised treatment plan to include both the stammering and any coexisting difficulty. To date, there have been no studies investigating the effectiveness of any approach treating children who stammer who also have additional difficulties. We would typically recommend the indirect component of Palin PCI (interaction and family strategies) as the initial package of therapy, followed by direct therapy for the language or phonology, or both, as well as the stammering, as appropriate. When a child has a diagnosis of SLI, ADHD or ASD we may have access to a specialist SLT within our service who is also working with the child. Therapy targeting his other difficulties is likely to be taking place alongside the therapy aimed at developing his fluency.

School or preschool liaison

The real-world environment of a young child who stammers is our key focus of intervention. In many cases it is sufficient to work with parents and families to make small changes to facilitate the child's fluency. We have worked with many parents who are in full-time employment and whose children attend full-time day care. It might be expected that in these cases intervention would be less effective as the child's contact with his parents is reduced and he has less exposure to the fluency-facilitating strategies. However, we have found that these children progress well, and working with the parents is sufficient to effect a positive outcome.

However, parents sometimes ask that preschool or school staff be given information about the child's stammering problem. With the parents' consent, we routinely send the school or preschool a copy of the report, which outlines the nature of the stammering problem, factors which may be contributing to it and the treatment recommendations. We may provide further specific information and advice as necessary, either by telephone contact, in written form or by visiting.

General knowledge about stammering tends to be limited, and even if staff have had experience of other children who stammer, this might not be relevant for this child.

It may be helpful to give information about why the child is stammering and what seems to affect it.

Preschool and school staff may be unsure about how they should respond to the child when he stammers. It is helpful to reassure them that it is fine to be sympathetic when they notice a child is struggling to speak, just as they would if a child were struggling with another task: 'Oh that was hard, wasn't it? Well done, you got there in the end.' Staff may also need specific advice on what to say if they want to help the child, or when just to listen. A general rule of thumb is that they should not feel under pressure to say the word for the child.

General advice can also be given on managing the child's stammering in the group context. Most preschools and schools are highly aware of the importance of turn-taking, which will be particularly helpful for the child who stammers. However, it may be appropriate to inform them that if the child who stammers is speaking at great length or monopolising turns it is appropriate to ask him to let others speak. Staff have sometimes reported that they are fearful of asking the child to stop talking, which can result in him unfairly dominating circle times or other group discussions.

Staff may also benefit from knowing specific strategies that the parents are using to facilitate the child's fluency, such as the use of pausing or using a slow rate of speech. It is important to have realistic expectations of people who are managing large groups of children. Monitoring our interaction style in a one-to-one setting may be a challenge, doing so with a class of children may seem impossible. However, some teachers have adopted a whole-class approach to fluency strategies, which is very helpful.

Palin PCI may be adapted for use with preschool staff and other key workers. If the child has a specific key worker or teacher who is willing and available for training, this can augment the therapy programme (see Chapter 10).

Staff may need to monitor other children's reactions to the child who stammers. Many young children seem blithely unaware of the differences in others, but sometimes there is a curiosity and a lack of inhibition about making a remark. There may be no malice or humiliation intended, just a desire for information: 'Why do you talk like that?', 'Why does he talk funny?' Staff can respond in a matter-of-fact way: 'He talks like that because it is hard for him to get some of his words out. He knows what he wants to say; it just takes him longer to say it. We can help him by waiting for him.' It is also important to watch for early signs of teasing, laughing at the child or mimicking him. Much to the surprise and horror of his parents and his teacher, one four-year-old child told us in his child assessment that the other children at school called him '*the but but but boy*'.

In-service training sessions to groups of preschool staff or schoolteachers can also be useful. They might include the following:

- A group brainstorm on the different types of stammering and any associated emotions
- A brainstorm on the various causes of stammering
- Some facts about stammering
- A brainstorm of what people can do to help when a child is stammering
- Useful preschool or classroom strategies
- A discussion on children's reactions to stammering, including teasing
- A question and answer session.

Onward referral

As previously mentioned, if a child has associated difficulties that require assessment or intervention, we refer on to other agencies in consultation with the parents.

Adapting Palin PCI

10

Structured therapy programmes can be useful clinical tools. They provide a step by step guide through the assessment and treatment process. However, a 'one size fits all' approach is unlikely to meet the needs of all children, and this is certainly true for a caseload of children who stammer. Most researchers and clinicians agree that no two children who stammer are the same and therefore each child will require treatment to be tailored to his specific needs.

Adapting Palin PCI for families with different cultural or linguistic backgrounds

Use of interpreters

In order to ensure that we are providing an equitable service to children and families from all backgrounds we often need interpreters to assist in assessment and therapy. At the MPC, we use professional interpreters who have been appropriately trained, rather than family members, in order to ensure that personal factors are not interfering with the information that is being exchanged.

When we are working on parents' styles of interaction, we always encourage them to speak in the language which they would usually use with the child. When this is other than English, we ask the interpreter to translate for us.

Cultural differences

Interpreters can also be invaluable in providing us with general information about a particular culture, such as attitudes to disability, roles of mothers and fathers, expectations of therapy. However, we are cautious of making generalisations about a culture, as each family will have its own unique set of attitudes and customs. We have found families themselves to be the most useful source of information about their cultural and personal styles.

We have found that some cultural groups find aspects of Palin PCI more challenging. If parents are not accustomed to the idea of playing with toys we may need to be creative in helping them to establish Special Times. We might suggest that they spend Special Times doing something the child enjoys, such as a special cooking activity or going to the park together.

Furthermore, there are also cultural differences with regard to use of eye contact, taking turns to speak, sleep regimens and so on. However, one of the strengths of Palin PCI is that it is based on the premise that parents instinctively know what helps their child, and are already doing this much of the time. Palin PCI helps them to do more. We are not asking them to stop doing something, or to start using a new and different style. This means that, whatever a parent's cultural or personal style, they will be developing the aspects of their interaction and management style in ways that they understand to be most helpful to their child. In this way Palin PCI is intrinsically culturally and personally sensitive to individual families' needs.

Adapting Palin PCI when only one parent is available

It is important that families have equal access to Palin PCI whatever their personal circumstances may be. When one parent is living away from home, perhaps working or studying abroad, we start therapy with the parent who is available and then arrange further input when the other parent is at home. If parents have separated or divorced, but are both caring for the child, we would ask them if they want to attend sessions together or separately. In the case of single-parent families, if there is a significant other carer, for example a new partner or a grandparent whom the parent wishes to include, we would invite them to participate in sessions. If the child is looked after by another person, such as a childminder, nanny or grandparent, we sometimes involve this person in the therapy.

Adapting Palin PCI when neither parent is available

Sometimes SLTs work in settings where there is no or limited access to parents. We would always encourage therapists to involve parents in the treatment of young children who stammer, for the reasons described earlier in Chapter 1. We can initially establish a child's level of vulnerability to persistence through a telephone conversation (see Chapter 2) if the parents are unable to attend for an initial 20-minute appointment. If a full assessment is recommended at this stage, the child assessment can take place in the preschool and then it may be possible to arrange a session with the parents for the case history and formulation. We have sometimes found that, once parents have attended the case history session, they have understood their role in the therapy process and are available to take part in the therapy programme. If this is not the case, the therapist now has a treatment plan, which may be implemented in alternative ways.

A home programme

- *Home programme record*
- *Special Times instruction sheet*
- *Special Times task sheet*
- *Interaction strategies handouts*
- *Family strategies handouts*

Following the case history session, we ask the parents to attend for a 90-minute session.

- We set up the Special Times with each parent, giving each of them a Special Times instruction sheet (see Appendix XII) and six copies of the Special Times task sheet (see Appendix XIII). We decide with each parent how many Special Times they will do each week and record this on their home programme record (see Appendix XXX).
- We ask the parents what they think the child needs in order to be more fluent and record this on the home programme record.
- We make a video of each parent playing with the child.
- We watch the video with each parent to identify up to three interaction strategies that they would like to do more of in order to help their child's fluency.
- We decide with each parent the order in which they will work on these targets and write the targets on the home programme record.
- We give the parents copies of the interaction strategies handouts (see Appendices XIV–XVIII) that are relevant to their chosen targets.
- We discuss with the parents the family strategies that were identified during the assessment and give them the relevant handouts (see Appendices XXI, XXII and XXIV–XXVII).
- We decide with them the order in which they will work on these strategies and write these on the home programme record.
- We ask the parents to spend the first week establishing the Special Times in their home routine, and then completing their task sheets.
- We ask the parents to telephone us at the end of the first week to discuss how they are getting on. Telephone calls are arranged for a specific day and time and this is written on the home programme record, together with the therapist's telephone number. We inform parents that the telephone calls are viewed in the same way as a clinic appointment and

therefore the therapist will make sure she is available at the arranged time for half an hour.

- We ask the parents to send, fax or email their task sheets to the therapist after the telephone call.

When the parents telephone at the end of the first week we discuss how they have managed with implementing Special Times and completing their task sheets. If they are satisfied that the routine is established, we ask them to read and complete the first interaction strategy handout at home and then try to implement the target during their Special Times in the following week.

At the end of the second week, the parents telephone to give feedback on their Special Times and we decide with them whether they will continue to practise the same interaction target for the next week, or whether they will add their next target. We also ask the parents to read and complete their first family strategy handout at home and then try out some of the suggestions. 'Building my child's confidence' (see Appendix XXI) is the first family strategy to be introduced.

For the next four weeks, the parents continue to do Special Times at home, implementing interaction and family strategies, as appropriate. They telephone us at the end of each week to discuss what has happened and then send, email or fax in their task sheets.

This phase of the home programme continues for six weeks, after which the parents continue to do their Special Times and implement the family strategies for a further period of six weeks (the consolidation period), sending in their task sheets but without the weekly telephone appointments. At the end of this phase, we review with the parents (either by telephone or in the clinic) the child's progress and decide on further management accordingly.

Interaction therapy with another adult

If the child attends a preschool and the parents are unavailable to attend the clinic for therapy or to do the home programme, we may consider working with a member of preschool or school staff. This method of adapting PCI has been used with children with speech and language difficulties in Early Years settings (Hulme, 2005). This approach is most appropriate if the child has a designated key worker who is available and willing to work with us. We then adapt the Palin PCI programme as follows.

- We discuss with the key worker the assessment findings and ask their views on what seems to help the child.

- We write down a list of things that the key worker will be aiming to help the child to do. For example, 'We want to help him to take it more slowly and to give himself more time to think about what he wants to say.'
- We discuss how those things will help the child's fluency.
- We make a video recording of the key worker playing with the child.
- We watch the video with the key worker and help them to identify times when they are helping the child to do the things on the list.
- We discuss with the key worker one target that they could do more of to further help the child's fluency. We may use the relevant interaction strategy handouts. These handouts may need to be adapted as they refer to 'my child'.
- We suggest to the key worker that they have special five-minute practice times with the child once a day when they will try to focus on the target to help his fluency.

We may also discuss with the key worker other strategies from the family strategies chapter which they could implement with the child, for example 'Building my child's confidence', 'Turn-taking', 'Dealing with feelings' and 'High standards'. The relevant handouts may be used as necessary

11

What Parents Say about Palin PCI and Summary

What the parents say

'The advice and guidance we received were very clearly and gently given. The results were extraordinary.'

(Mother of Joe, aged three)

'The first great help was the fact that Raja felt at ease straight away and was able to confide in the therapist about school and bullying. All parties involved were then able to deal with the situation immediately and the change was noticeable straight away. The second great help was to be told again that it wasn't our fault, us, parents. The therapist helped us define strategies and games to help Raja, making us understand how to work with him and for him, how to deal with various situations. It was a lot of work, being involved but the results were immediate again.

The stammer changed from really worrying, to being able to handle it, to quite fine actually, to none at all.

Now, we just stick to the routine, in an easy way, not being stressed about not doing it one day, just helping Raja with some 'Special Times', Bus Talking and lots of praise and self-confidence building.

The therapist is always available for help and it is reassuring to know that someone is there to help, reassure and just speak about stammering.'

(Mother of Raja, aged four)

'The assessment was great, really interesting, thorough and Holly really enjoyed it too. In the therapy the use of cameras and feedback was fascinating and it was nice to hear about what we did that was positive, as well as what we could do to help Holly.

Holly enjoyed the whole process and at no time felt stigmatised or upset about her speech problem and this was in part due to your professional and reassuring and lovely manner with her. It was a very non-clinical and fun approach for her.

The 'Special Time' sessions were predictably hard to fit in, which made me realise how little quality one-to-one time my kids actually get from me, but we did the sessions and it was really nice.

I learnt how hard it is to change my fast speech or ways of communicating and that it needs lots of mindfulness and practice.

I suspect that if her problem emerges again I will know how to help her from the lessons and therapy sessions.'

(Mother of Holly, aged five)

'We have been very impressed with the way you have tailored what you offer to what we have needed. We feel very lucky that we have access to you.'

(Father of Lucy, aged three)

'Before we started the therapy, I was worried about a number of things. Mostly, that Kai's stammer would affect his experience of growing up and, ultimately, it would mean that he would not have a happy life. I was worried that people would make fun of him and would not play with him and I was worried that this might make him introverted and shy and mean that he was not able to interact in social situations. I did not want Kai to be unhappy and I was very nervous that it was something that we could not do anything about and that maybe it might get worse.

When we first went for the assessment, I felt a sense of relief that we were in an environment where people understood and accepted that Kai did have a stammer. We had spoken about it to other people before we came for therapy and everybody had said that it was something that Kai would grow out of and that we should not worry, it would be fine. To finally be among people that not only understood how we all felt, but also could offer some help in managing Kai's speech was really great. It was a safe space for us all to look at what was happening and put a plan of action in place as to what we were going to do. It has helped us to all work together and become more of a unit – and that includes our daughter, Kai's sister.

I think that, ironically, the speech therapy has encouraged Kai's language skills so that he seems more able to express himself than many other children I have met.'

(Mother of Kai, aged three)

'When, at two and a half, our happy, verbose little boy began to stammer we put it down to a stage that he was going through. By three he was blocking and grimacing when he tried to talk and we were desperately trying to find the right help for him. For us the most difficult time was the period of nine months or so when we were waiting to be seen. It seemed to us that his fluency was deteriorating

with every week that passed and we worried greatly about whether the delay in treatment would cause long-term damage to his speech. It was very hard to watch him struggle with his words and be unable to help him.

From the outset the therapist gave us a very clear explanation of how the therapy was structured and what each step was designed to achieve. That approach gave us a level of understanding that enabled us to feel empowered and incredibly positive about the therapy.

Before coming to the Michael Palin Centre our experience of speech therapy for children had been of a rather demanding, mechanical, physical process, and we were very concerned about how such a little boy would cope with those pressures. Nothing could be further from our experience of therapy at the Michael Palin Centre. Their holistic, family-based therapy has meant that our son did not even realise that he was having speech therapy. Much of the therapy, such as building a child's confidence through praise and helping a sensitive child to deal with the world, is of wider application. Our family has benefited enormously from the support and practical advice given by the therapists. We feel incredibly fortunate to have had access to the therapy and our son, now seven and a half, no longer stammers.'

(Mother of Charlie, aged seven and a half)

'Archie has never attended any sort of speech therapy before so I was little apprehensive as I did not know what to expect. I have had concerns over his speech, and always felt that he would grow out of it like his older brother, but as time progressed this did not appear to be happening.

At the start of the first session I thought Archie initially spoke quite clearly and I thought maybe I had over-stated his problem. But as the session progressed it was clear that his stammer was quite severe (33 per cent). I felt guilty that maybe I should have reacted sooner and got professional advice.

We are now into the third week of our programme. I was surprised at first as to the focus of therapy. I thought the emphasis would be on the way he spoke and his breathing. But I understand that maybe the key to unlocking his stammering is to create an environment where his emotional needs are met. He is a sensitive boy and maybe his reaction to his busy, hectic lifestyle has affected his speech. The therapy has also highlighted the way we as parents interact with him.

I feel positive that with all the support, at home, at the centre and from his teacher at school, he will overcome his stammering.'

(Mother of Archie, aged four)

Summary

Palin PCI is an evidence-based programme for the assessment and management of early stammering. We have developed the approach over a number of years and it combines indirect and direct methods, using interaction, family and child strategies to develop a child's fluency. Parents and others in the child's environment are key to implementing the programme. The philosophy and techniques of the approach can also be used with children with other speech, language and communication difficulties.

We hope you have found this book useful in further developing your knowledge and skills in working with early stammering, and we encourage therapists to attend a Palin PCI training course to consolidate what they have already learnt.

Appendices

I Initial screening form

II Information and advice for parents

III Summary Chart

IV Child assessment booklet

V Assessment of stammering

VI Child assessment booklet: Scott

VII Child assessment booklet: Khaled

VIII Case history

IX Summary chart: Scott

X Summary chart: Khaled

XI General facts about stammering

XII Special Times instruction sheet

XIII Special Times task sheet

XIV 'Letting my child take the lead in play' handout

XV 'Keeping things simple' handout

XVI 'Balancing comments and questions' handout

XVII 'My rate of talking and use of pauses' handout

XVIII 'Eye contact and talking' handout

XIX Questions for the SLT to ask in Palin PCI sessions

XX Special Times task sheet: Scott

XXI 'Building my child's confidence' handout

XXII 'Openness about stammering' handout

XXIII Praise log

XXIV 'Taking turns to talk' handout

XXV 'Helping my child to deal with his feelings' handout

XXVI 'The child whose standards are too high' handout

XXVII 'Managing my child's behaviour' handout

XXVIII Tortoise Talking practice chart

XXIX Bus Talking practice chart

XXX Palin PCI home programme record

Initial screening form 1 of 2

APPENDIX I

Child's name ______________________

Date of birth ______________ Age ______________

Language spoken ______________ Date ______________

Parents' description of the problem

What does he do when he stammers?

- ☐ Does he repeat whole words, eg, *but but but*?
- ☐ Does he repeat parts of words, eg, *b-b-but*?
- ☐ Does he stretch out sounds, eg, *mmmmum*?
- ☐ Does he get stuck on a sound and nothing comes out?
- ☐ Does he do anything else with his face or body when he stammers?
- ☐ Does he give up on trying to say it?

Do you think he is aware of it?

____

Do you think he is worried about it?

____

On a scale of 0 to 7 where 0 is normal and 7 is very severe, how severe is the stammering?

0 1 2 3 4 5 6 7

When did he start stammering?

____

Has it changed since then? In what way?

____

When is it better and when is it worse?

____

On a scale of 0 to 7, where 0 is not at all worried and 7 is extremely worried, where are you now?

0 1 2 3 4 5 6 7

If he/she is talking to you and stammers, what do you do or say to try and help?

____

____

____

Family history

	Mother	*Father*
Has either of you ever stammered?		
Do you still?		
Did any blood relative on either side of the family ever stammer?		
Do they still?		

Other speech, language, literacy problems

Does your child have any other speech or language difficulties now?

Do you think his language skills are better than those of other children of his age?

Any other issues we should be aware of?

Management

☐ Advice & Monitoring ☐ Child Assessment & Case History

Information and advice for parents 1 of 2

APPENDIX II

Fluency is a skill which gradually develops. Many children are hesitant in their speech as they learn new words, how to pronounce them and how to string words into sentences. When a child learns to walk, he may wobble, stumble and fall, especially in the early stages. Stumbling over sounds and words is a natural part of the process of learning to talk.

Parents do not cause stammering.

Four out of five young children who stammer will recover. There are a number of 'risk factors' which indicate which children are more likely to persist in stammering.

The children who are most likely to recover from stammering are those who:

1. Are already showing signs of getting better
2. Don't have any relatives who stammer
3. Aren't aware or worried about their speech
4. Don't have any other problems with speaking
5. Don't have advanced language skills
6. Have been stammering for less than a year
7. Have parents who are not worried about the stammering.

Some advice for parents

There are ways that you could help your child to be more fluent. You are probably doing some of these already, but there may be some new ideas.

- If a child gives himself time, he can think and plan what he is trying to say and he can co-ordinate the movements involved in speaking. Many children rush in to speak. You could try to set the pace for your child by trying to model pauses before you speak and using an unhurried rate.

- We all ask questions, and when a child is asked a question, he is expected to respond. His ability to answer fluently will depend on how difficult the question is and how good his language skills are. Parents can help their child to answer more fluently by:

  1. Avoiding questions which are too complicated for your child
  2. Giving him plenty of time to think of and give his reply
  3. Avoiding asking another question before he has had time to answer the first one.

- When we are in a group, we often overlap or interrupt each other. It can be harder for a child who stammers if he is rushing to finish what he wants to say before someone else butts in or if he is rushing to interrupt someone else. You could help your child by ensuring that everybody listens to each other and nobody interrupts the speaker. He will then feel able to take his time and this can help him to be more fluent. It's also important to remember to keep things fair – other family members should have their say, as well as the child who stammers.
- If you can give your child some one-to-one 'quality' time, this may help him as he will have your undivided attention and there is no need to rush. In a busy family lifestyle, you may find it useful to have a brief, regular slot with each child.

Summary Chart

APPENDIX III

Child's name ______________________ Date ____________

Stammering & Social Communication Skills				
% ss	*Parent rating*			Child's awareness/concern
Type of stammering	*WWR*	*PWR*	*Prol.*	*Blocking*
Time since onset	*< 6mths*	*<12mths*	*>12mths*	
Pattern of change	*Better*	*Same*	*Worse*	
Parents' levels of concern				

Child's awareness/concern	
Talking at length/turn-taking	
Reduced eye contact	
Reduced concentration	

Linguistic	
History of delayed speech/language development	
Reduced receptive skills	
Reduced expressive skills	
Word finding difficulty	
Speech sound difficulty	
Advanced language skills	
Mismatch within/between speech/language skills	
Managing two languages	

Physiological	
Family history of stammering	
Co-ordination	
Tiredness	
Birth history	
Health	
Rapid bursts/rate of speech	

Psychological	
Reduced confidence	
High standards	
Increased sensitivity	
Anxious/worrier	
Difficulties coping with change	
Reaction to stammering	

Environmental	
Turn-taking in family	
Behaviour management	
Routines	
Openness about stammering	
Preschool/school issues	
Pace of life	

What does this child need?
1
2
3

Interaction strategies	Helpful	Evidence of		Potential target	
		Mother	Father	Mother	Father
Following child's lead in play					
Letting child solve problems					
More comments than questions					
Complexity of questions at child's level					
Language is appropriate to child's level					
Language is semantically contingent on child's focus					
Repetition, expansion, rephrasing					
Time to initiate, respond, finish					
Rate of input when compared with child's rate					
Use of pausing					
Using eye contact, position, touch, humour and/or surprise					
Praise and encouragement					

Family strategies	
Special Times	
Managing two languages	
Openness about stammering	
Building confidence	
Turn-taking	
Dealing with feelings	
High standards	
Sleep	
Behaviour management	
Routines	
Pace of life	
Emerging issues	

Child strategies	
Rate reduction	
Pausing to think	
Easy onset	
Being more concise	
Eye contact/ focus of attention	

Other	
Language/phonology therapy	
School/preschool liaison	
Onward referral	

Child assessment booklet 1 of 5

Child assessment synopsis

Child's name ______________________ Date of birth ______________

Date ______________ Age ______________ Clinician ______________

Stammering

Type

Percentage

Awareness / concern

Rate of speech

Receptive language

Informal

Formal

Expressive language

Informal

Formal

Word finding

Speech sound development

Social skills

Attention control / listening

Eye contact

Animation

Turn-taking / talking at length

Separation

Co-operation

Anxiety

Other comments

Transcription

Assessment of stammering

Percentage stammered syllables	$\frac{\text{Total no. of stammered syllables}}{\text{Total no. of syllables spoken}} \times 100 =$ %SS		
Whole-word repetitions	number of repetitions		
Part-word repetitions	number of repetitions		
Prolongations	length	change in pitch / volume	
Blocks	length		
Other			
Facial tension	eyes	mouth	other
Body movements	hands	feet	other
Disrupted breathing	gasping	ingressive	end of breath
Awareness	☐ Child says, *'I can't say it'* ☐ Child gives up ☐ Child looks away during struggle ☐ Your instinct		
Avoidance	☐ Changes word ☐ Avoids word ☐ Avoids situations ☐ Uses fillers		
Speech rate	moderate / generally rapid / rapid bursts		
Severity rating			
Other observations			

The child's perspective

School

Do you go to preschool/school?

Do you like it there?

What is good/what do you like doing?

What don't you like doing?

What is your teacher like? or, Tell me about your teacher.

Do you like her? Why? Why not?

Does she get cross? With you? Why?

Do you have friends? Tell me their names.

What do you like doing with your friends?

Are there any children who are nasty to you?

What do they do/say?

How does that make you feel?

What do you do when they are nasty?

Do you tell anybody?

Home

Who lives with you at home?

Tell me about your mummy.

What do you like doing with her?

Tell me about your daddy.

What do you like doing with him?

Tell me about your brother(s).

What do you like doing with him?

Tell me about your sister(s).

What do you like doing with her?

What don't you like doing at home?

Speech

Why did mummy/daddy bring you here today?

How are you getting on with your talking?

Is it sometimes hard to talk?

What happens?

How does it make you feel?

If appropriate, therapist models WWR, PWR, prolongations and blocking.

When it is hard to talk, can you do anything to make it better?

What do mummy or daddy do to help you with your talking?

Would you like some help with talking?

General

What is the best thing that ever happened to you?

What is the worst thing that ever happened to you?

What do you do if you have a problem?

Let's pretend I can do magic and I could change something about you. What would you want me to change?

Assessment of stammering 1 of 5

The audio- or video-recorded speech sample collected during the child assessment is transcribed and the stammering episodes identified. It is then analysed to:

Step 1: Transcription
Step 2: Identification of stammering episodes
Step 3: Calculation of % SS
Step 4: Description of stammering behaviours
Step 5: Severity rating

- Calculate the percentage of stammered syllables
- Describe the types of stammering behaviours observed
- Obtain a severity rating.

Step 1: Transcription

We do a written transcription of the speech sample on the Transcription sheet in the child assessment booklet (Appendix IV). When the child has described approximately ten '*What's Wrong?*' pictures (LDA, 1988), this produces about 300 syllables of his speech, which is a reasonably sized sample to capture a child's level of fluency (Conture, 2001; Guitar, 2006).

Step 2: Identifying each episode of stammering

We then identify the episodes of stammering and mark them on the transcript. We underline each syllable where there is an episode of stammering.

The following behaviours are counted as stammering:

- *Single-syllable, whole-word repetitions*

  For example:
  - I-I (one repetition)
  - and-and-and (two repetitions)
  - it-it-it-it (three repetitions)

  Only single-syllable, whole-word repetitions are counted as stammering. They are recorded on the transcription with the whole word written out the number of times it has been repeated.

- *Part-word repetitions*

  Part-word repetitions include repetitions of sounds and syllables. For example:
  - c-c-c-cat (three repetitions)
  - mu-mu-mu-mu-mummy (four repetitions)

As with whole-word repetitions, the number of times a sound or syllable is repeated is reflected in the transcription. If there is evidence of changes in vowel quality we transcribe this phonetically. For example:

– bə- bə-because

- *Sound prolongations*

  We record sound prolongations on the transcription by writing down the : symbol after the sound that has been prolonged. For example:

  – m:ummy, mumm:y, mu:mmy

  For some children sound prolongations are accompanied by an increase in loudness or pitch. This can be marked on the transcription by the use of a ↑. For example:

  – mu:↑mmy

- *Blocking*

  Blocks are marked by circling the sound which has been blocked. For example:

  – (b)all, po(t)ato, (a)pple

Some episodes of blocking, for example laryngeal blocking, may be silent and therefore not perceptible on an audio recording. If a video recording is not being made, it is important to make a note of such behaviour 'live' during the assessment.

We do not count the following as episodes of stammering:

- Multi-syllabic whole words that are repeated, for example, 'because-because'
- Interjections, for example, 'she is um cooking with a hammer'; 'I cook with a uh uh you know a spoon'
- Phrase repetitions, for example, 'the girl-the girl-the girl is painting with a carrot'; 'a duck in the-in the boat'
- Revisions, for example, 'she wants a bi- a cake'; 'the bike's got cir- got square wheels'.

However, we make a note of the above behaviours as they may be an indication that a child has language formulation problems or needs to give himself more time to generate his ideas or to find a specific word.

Step 3: Calculate the percentage of stammered syllables

When the transcription is completed, we can then calculate the percentage of stammered syllables.

The percentage of stammered syllables is calculated by:

(a) Counting the total number of stammered syllables

(b) Counting the total number of syllables spoken in the sample. We count every syllable spoken apart from the repeated syllables in an episode of stammering. For example:

my-my bike = 2 syllables spoken
ca-ca-ca-carrot = 2 syllables spoken
my bike-my bike = 4 syllables spoken
because-because = 4 syllables spoken

(c) Using the following formula:

$$\frac{\text{total no. of stammered syllables}}{\text{total no. of syllables spoken}} \times 100$$

	Stamm. syll	Syll. spoken
The bike's g-g-g-got square wheels	1	5
They supposed to be r:ound	1	6
I ride my-my bike in the (p)ark	2	7
My bike hasn't got square wheels, mine are round	0	10
The water's going going over the bridge, that's not right	0	14
um um the (g)irl is the girl is painting w:ith a carrot	2	12
I-I-I paint with a p-p-(p)aintbrush	2	6
The duck um um is w:earing b-b-b-boots	2	6
Duck's (d)on't w:ear boots, chi- no, people wear boots	2	9
I wear my boots when it's rai- when it's muddy	0	10
He's s: he's s: he's s:tirring with a h-h-h-(h)ammer	2	9
My dad my dad doesn't s:tir with a um um h-h-h-hammer, he s:tirs with a spoon	3	16
You use a hammer to bang um um nails	0	8

Total no. of stammered syllables = 17

Total no. of syllables spoken = 118

Percentage of stammered syllables: $\frac{17}{118} \times 100 = 14.4$ %SS

Step 4: Description of the types of stammering behaviours observed

Note the types of stammering behaviours observed on the 'Assessment of stammering form'

Once we have calculated the percentage of stammered syllables, we make a note of the different types of stammering behaviours (ie, WWR, PWR, prolongations and blocking) identified during the recorded speech sample and observed during the rest of the assessment session. These are recorded on the 'Assessment of stammering form' (page 3 of the 'Child assessment booklet', Appendix IV). We also note down the number of times a word, sound or syllable is typically repeated in whole-word and part-word repetitions. We also give an approximate estimate of the length of prolongations and blocking.

Other

We have included an 'Other' category which may be used to describe any other behaviours noted, such as repeated use of fillers or starters, insertion of additional sounds at the beginning of words, changes in pitch or loudness, clicks, etc.

Facial tension/body movements

We make a note of any signs of tension or struggling behaviour, for example, foot-tapping, head movements, shoulder tension, nostrils flaring, eyes blinking.

Disrupted breathing

We comment on any signs of disrupted breathing. For example, the child may be talking on an ingressive airstream, gasping for breath or running out of breath before finishing his sentences.

Awareness

A child does not always express awareness of the stammer when we ask him about it directly, but he may show signs of awareness during the speech sample or the rest of the assessment session, such as saying 'I can't say it', giving up or looking away during moments of stammering. We may also just have an instinct that a child is aware.

Avoidance

Although word avoidance is less common in young children who stammer, it can sometimes be apparent in this age group. We may notice that a child starts to say a word, begins to stammer and then changes it. For example:

- 'I like eating ca-ca…biscuits'
- 'How old are you?' '(f)i-(f)i…I'm five years old.'

In addition, a child may be using interjections or fillers such as 'uh', 'er', 'um' as a way of postponing saying a word they anticipate stammering on. If we notice any signs of word avoidance we ask the child whether they ever change or avoid words because of their stammer.

Speech rate

We do not formally measure a child's rate of speech during the assessment but make a subjective judgement about his rate during different speaking tasks. We note whether the child shows a slow or moderate rate, is generally rapid or speaks in rapid bursts.

Step 5: Severity of stammering

A severity rating can be obtained using the Yairi and Ambrose severity rating scale (Yairi & Ambrose, 2005). As a published outcome measure, this may be useful in clinical audit or research studies, as well as being a helpful clinical tool. It is an eight-point scale ranging from 0 = normal speech to 7 = very severe stammering. The numerical value is calculated from the percentage of stammered syllables and the average duration of the five longest stammering episodes observed, as well as the presence of tension and secondary behaviours.

The information from the 'Assessment of stammering form' is then summarised on the child assessment synopsis form (see Appendix IV) on the front of the 'Child assessment booklet'.

Child assessment booklet: Scott

APPENDIX VI

Child assessment synopsis

Child's name *Scott* Date of birth

Date Age *3 yrs 2 mths* Clinician *AN*

Stammering

Type *WWR 3 repetitions PWR 3 repetitions Prolongations 3 secs Blocking*

Percentage *9.8%*

Awareness / concern *'I can't say my words'*

Rate of speech *Rapid bursts*

Receptive language

Informal *Understood conversation language & instructions*

Formal *Standard Score 118 Age equivalent 6 yrs 4 mths*

Expressive language

Informal *Very verbal. Sophisticated vocabulary & grammatical structures*

Formal *Vocabulary age equivalent 6.5 yrs. Grammar age equivalent 6 yrs*

Word finding *NAD*

Speech sound development *NAD*

Social skills

Attention control / listening *Very good*

Eye contact *Looked away during blocks*

Animation *NAD*

Turn-taking / talking at length *Waited for turn, then took lengthy turns*

Separation

Co-operation *Excellent*

Anxiety *Wanted to know if he got things right*

Other comments

Showed urgency, eg, with formboards

Lined pictures up carefully

Child assessment booklet: Khaled

APPENDIX VII

Child assessment synopsis

Child's name *Khaled* Date of birth

Date Age *5 yrs 1 mth* Clinician *EK*

Stammering

Type *WWR 2 repetitions PWR 4 repetitions 1 Prolongation*

Percentage *6%*

Awareness / concern *None apparent*

Rate of speech *Rapid*

Receptive language

Informal *Understood conversation language & instructions*

Formal *Standard Score 101 Age equivalent 5 yr 2 mths*

Expressive language

Informal *Appropriate vocabulary & grammatical structures*

Formal *Vocabulary age equivalent 5 yr. Grammar age equivalent 5 yr*

Word finding *NAD*

Speech sound development *Delayed phonology. Stopping, cluster reduction. Intelligibility affected at times, especially with rapid rate.*

Social skills

Attention control / listening *Appropriate*

Eye contact *Appropriate*

Animation *NAD*

Turn-taking / talking at length *Appropriate*

Separation

Co-operation *Excellent*

Anxiety *None evident*

Other comments

Case history

Biographical details

Family name ______________________________

First name(s) ______________________________

Male/female ________ Date of birth ______________ Age on date of interview ________

Home address ______________________________

____

Postcode ______________ Tel ______________

Mother's name ______________________________

Address (if different) ______________________________

Telephone ______________________________

Father's name ______________________________

Address (if different) ______________________________

Telephone ______________________________

First language ______________ Interpreter ______________

School/preschool ______________________________

Address ______________________________

Head teacher ______________ Telephone ______________

GP ______________________________

Address ______________________________

Interviewer ______________ **Date** ______________

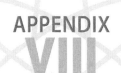

PRIVATE AND CONFIDENTIAL

Presenting problem

Are there any other problems apart from the stammering that you are worried about?

If so, which is your main concern at the moment?

What does he do when he stammers?
(Repeats whole words eg, but but but? Repeats parts of words eg, b-b-but? Stretches sounds eg, mmmmum? Gets stuck on a sound and nothing comes out? Does he do anything else with his face or body when he stammers? Does he do anything to try to hide it?)

Does he avoid words? Situations? Does he ever give up saying something?

Do you think he is aware of it? Concerned about it? What gives that impression?

Do you think his stammer affects his confidence?

Does he seem to have any strategies for managing his stammer?

When did he start stammering?

Was there anything in particular going on in his life at that time?
(eg, changes in preschool, school, birth of a sibling, family moving, other family changes or events?)

Did it start gradually or suddenly?

Has it changed since then? In what way?

When is the stammering worse? When does it happen the most?

When is the stammering better? When does it happen the least?

Do you talk about the stammering with your child?

What do you do or say when your child stammers?

Parents:

Siblings:

What seems to help him most?

On a scale of 0–7 where 0 is normal and 7 is very severe, how severe is his stammer?

Mother	0	1	2	3	4	5	6	7
Father	0	1	2	3	4	5	6	7

On a scale of 0–7 where 0 is not at all worried and 7 is extremely worried, where are you now?

Mother	0	1	2	3	4	5	6	7
Father	0	1	2	3	4	5	6	7

Has your child had therapy before? What happened?

What are you hoping for today?

Communication

Does he have any other problems with communication, speech or language?

Does he speak as well as other children of the same age?

Does he speak clearly?

What is his rate of speech like?

Bi/multilingual: does your child speak more than one language?

If so, what language is spoken at home?

Which does he use the most?

Are there any differences in his stammering in the languages?

Health and development

How is your child's general health?

Have you ever had concerns about his hearing?

Has his hearing ever been tested?

What is his concentration like?

Is he fidgety or restless?

What is his co-ordination like?

Eating and sleeping

Are there any problems with eating or mealtimes?
(If so, what? How currently managed? Do both parents agree? What helps most?)

What about sleeping?

What time does he go to bed?

When does he wake?

Does he sleep through the night?

Does he stay in his own bed?

Do you think he gets enough sleep?

Personality

How would you describe your child's personality?

Would you say that he is sensitive, or not particularly? *(examples)*

How does he react if he gets something wrong or makes a mistake? *(examples)*

Does he like to please?

Does he worry, or not particularly? *(examples)*

Does he get upset easily, or not particularly? *(examples)*

Who does he take after?

Does he have a temper?
(How does he show his temper? Which situations trigger it? Is it an issue at school?)

How do you deal with it?

How does he cope with changes, new places and experiences?

Is he a child who likes routines?

How is he doing in terms of developing independence?

Child's relationships

How does your child get on with other children?

Does he have friends? Does he see them outside preschool/school?

Is he ever teased? Is he bullied? Does he get into fights?

Names and ages of brothers and sisters:

How do they get on?

How does he manage during family conversations?

Family history

	Mother	Father	Other family members
Ever stammered?			
Still stammer?			
Had therapy?			

What was the outcome?

Family relationships

How long have you been together/married?

Have you had any separations?

(Can you tell me a bit about what happened? How did your child cope with the changes?)

How would you say you get on as a couple?

One-parent families:

What contact does your child have with the other parent?

Who has full parental responsibility?

Have either of you started new relationships?

How does your child feel about these issues at the moment?

Do you have any concerns?

Schooling

How did your child first cope with going to preschool or school?

Do you have any concerns about his schooling? Are any changes planned?

What feedback do you get from staff?

Do you think he needs extra support? Does he have an Individual Education Plan?

Are the teachers concerned about his stammer?

What do his teachers do when he stammers?

Behaviour management

What do you do when he is naughty or needs discipline?

Do you both manage this in the same way? Are you consistent?

How does he react?

Is there anything that is difficult to manage at the moment?

Developmental history

Were there any complications during the pregnancy or birth?

Was he a full-term baby? What was his birth weight?

Were there any difficulties with feeding or other complications?

Were there any early difficulties during infancy?

When did he start to walk? When did he say his first words?

When did he say his first simple sentences?

When did he come out of nappies?

Were there any developmental problems?

Is there anything else you think we should know?

Summary of issues

Physiological

Speech and language

Environmental

Psychological

Management

Summary Chart: Scott

APPENDIX IX

Child's name *Scott* Date ____________

Stammering & Social Communication Skills

% ss *9.8%* Parent rating *Ma 7 Fa 6*	
Type of stammering WWR ✓ PWR ✓ Prol. ✓ Blocking ✓	
Time since onset < 6mths <12mths >12mths *12 months*	
Pattern of change Better Same Worse ✓	
Parents' levels of concern *Both 6*	

Child's awareness/concern *Aware & worried*	
Talking at length/turn-taking	
Reduced eye contact *during blocks*	
Reduced concentration	

Physiological

Family history of stammering	✓
Co-ordination	
Tiredness	
Birth history	
Health	
Rapid bursts/rate of speech	✓

Linguistic

History of delayed speech/language development	
Reduced receptive skills	
Reduced expressive skills	
Word finding difficulty	
Speech sound difficulty	
Advanced language skills	✓
Mismatch within/between speech/language skills	
Managing two languages	

Psychological

Reduced confidence	✓
High standards	✓
Increased sensitivity	✓
Anxious/worrier	✓
Difficulties coping with change	
Reaction to stammering	✓

Environmental

Turn-taking in family	✓
Behaviour management	
Routines	
Openness about stammering	✓
Preschool/school issues	
Pace of life	

What does this child need?

1 *To take pressure off himself by allowing more time, using shorter, simpler utterances and lower standards.*

2 *He needs to be able to express his feelings.*

3 *He needs a system of turn-taking with his sister.*

Interaction strategies	Helpful	Evidence of Mother	Evidence of Father	Potential target Mother	Potential target Father
Following child's lead in play	✓	✓	✓	✓	
Letting child solve problems					
More comments than questions	✓	✓	✓		
Complexity of questions at child's level	✓	✓	✓		
Language is appropriate to child's level	✓	✓	✓		
Language is semantically contingent on child's focus	✓	✓	✓		
Repetition, expansion, rephrasing					
Time to initiate, respond, finish	✓	✓	✓	✓	✓
Rate of input when compared with child's rate	✓	✓	✓		✓
Use of pausing	✓	✓	✓	✓	✓
Using eye contact, position, touch, humour and/or surprise	✓	✓	✓	✓	
Praise and encouragement	✓	✓	✓		

Family strategies	
Special Times	✓
Managing two languages	
Openness about stammering	✓
Building confidence	✓
Turn-taking	✓
Dealing with feelings	✓
High standards	✓
Sleep	
Behaviour management	
Routines	
Pace of life	
Emerging issues	

Child strategies	
Rate reduction	✓
Pausing to think	✓
Easy onset	
Being more concise	
Eye contact/ focus of attention	

Other	
Language/phonology therapy	
School/preschool liaison	
Onward referral	

Summary Chart: Khaled

APPENDIX X

Child's name *Khaled* Date ______________

Stammering & Social Communication Skills

% ss *6%*	Parent rating *Ma 3*
Type of stammering	WWR ✓ PWR ✓ Prol. ✓ Blocking
Time since onset	<6mths <12mths >12mths ✓
Pattern of change	Better Same ✓ Worse
Parents' levels of concern	*6*

Child's awareness/concern *Unaware*	
Talking at length/turn-taking	
Reduced eye contact	
Reduced concentration	

Physiological

Family history of stammering	✓
Co-ordination	✓
Tiredness	✓
Birth history	
Health	
Rapid bursts/rate of speech	✓

Psychological

Reduced confidence	✓
High standards	
Increased sensitivity	
Anxious/worrier	
Difficulties coping with change	
Reaction to stammering	

Linguistic

History of delayed speech/language development	
Reduced receptive skills	
Reduced expressive skills	
Word finding difficulty	
Speech sound difficulty	✓
Advanced language skills	
Mismatch within/between speech/language skills	✓
Managing two languages	✓

Environmental

Turn-taking in family	
Behaviour management	✓
Routines	
Openness about stammering	✓
Preschool/school issues	
Pace of life	

What does this child need?

1 *Khaled needs to give himself more time.*

2 *He needs to develop enough sleep to ensure that he is not tired.*

3 *He needs to develop his phonological skills.*

Interaction strategies	Helpful	Evidence of: Mother	Evidence of: Father	Potential target: Mother	Potential target: Father
Following child's lead in play	✓	✓		✓	
Letting child solve problems	✓				
More comments than questions	✓	✓			
Complexity of questions at child's level	✓	✓			
Language is appropriate to child's level	✓	✓			
Language is semantically contingent on child's focus	✓	✓			
Repetition, expansion, rephrasing	✓	✓		✓	
Time to initiate, respond, finish	✓	✓		✓	
Rate of input when compared with child's rate	✓	✓		✓	
Use of pausing	✓	✓		✓	
Using eye contact, position, touch, humour and/or surprise	✓	✓			
Praise and encouragement	✓	✓			

Family strategies	
Special Times	✓
Managing two languages	✓
Openness about stammering	
Building confidence	✓
Turn-taking	
Dealing with feelings	
High standards	
Sleep	✓
Behaviour management	✓
Routines	
Pace of life	
Emerging issues	

Child strategies	
Rate reduction	✓
Pausing to think	✓
Easy onset	
Being more concise	
Eye contact/ focus of attention	

Other	
Language/phonology therapy	✓
School/preschool liaison	
Onward referral	

General facts about stammering

APPENDIX XI

- Stammering has been around for centuries and, throughout history, many famous people have stammered, such as King George VI, Marilyn Monroe, Winston Churchill and, more recently, Rowan Atkinson, Bruce Willis and Tiger Woods.
- It occurs across the world and it is more common in boys than girls.
- Stammering tends to start between the ages of two and five, at a time when speech and language are developing.
- Research has shown that about five per cent of children start to stammer and one per cent continue to stammer into adult life. That means that approximately four out of five children will overcome the difficulty. Research is helping us work out which children are most likely to persist and what sorts of therapy may help.
- Stammering is a complicated problem because there is no single cause of stammering and no simple cure.

Multifactorial model

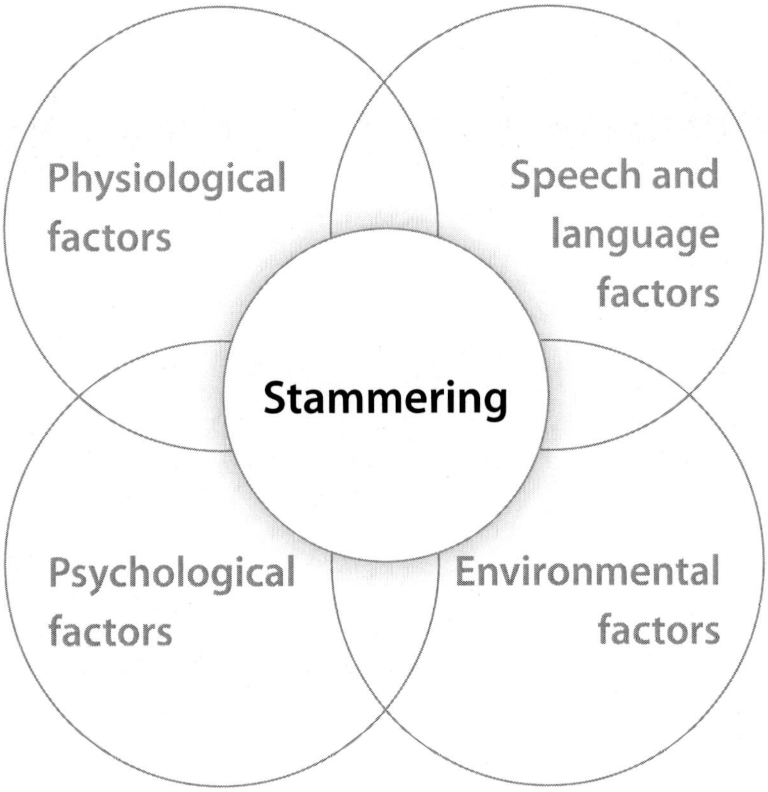

Special Times instruction sheet

Special Times last for five minutes only and should not be extended. Before you start, let your child choose the activity, toy or game. We don't want this to be reading a book, playing on a computer or a games console, watching TV or playing a lively outdoor game. When your child has decided what he wants to do, go somewhere where you won't be disturbed and deal with any obvious distractions such as the television or your telephone.

Play with your child for the five minutes, giving him your undivided attention and focusing on what he is saying rather than how he is saying it. When the time is up, write about your Special Time on the task sheet, making a note of what you did, and how you felt it went. Afterwards you can return to the activity with your child, but this is no longer part of Special Time.

If you have other children, it's a good idea to give them their own regular special times on an individual basis as well.

Special Times task sheet

APPENDIX XIII

Name of parent ______________________

Name of child ______________________

Number of Special Times ______________________

Targets for Special Times ______________________

DATE	ACTIVITY	COMMENTS ABOUT THE TARGETS

IN ONE SENTENCE, WRITE DOWN WHAT YOU HAVE LEARNT FROM THIS WEEK'S ACTIVITIES

'Letting my child take the lead in play' handout 1 of 2

APPENDIX XIV

Think

When I am playing with my child, who is usually in charge of the play? Is it my child or is it me?

Why might it be helpful to allow my child to take the lead in play?

What do I need to 'do more of', or 'do differently', in order to let my child lead the play?

Why we may be tempted to take charge of the child's play:

- If the child is sitting there not doing much
- If the activity is quite difficult and it is hard to watch a child struggle to do something
- Because we want to teach the child something
- Because we quite like to get our own way!

Why might it be helpful to allow my child to take the lead in play?

- It will help to keep the play at the child's level. He'll be choosing what he wants to do and this means he's less likely to be putting himself under pressure to do something which is too hard for him.
- It will help to keep the play at the child's pace – he can do things as quickly or slowly as he likes and he won't feel the need to try to keep up with somebody else.
- There will be more freedom for the child since he won't be following the adult's way of doing things.
- There is more opportunity for the child to develop:
  - — Problem-solving skills
  - — Play skills
  - — Imagination
  - — Self-confidence

What do I need to 'do more of' or 'do differently' in order to let my child lead the play?

STOP! LOOK! LISTEN! (not just useful for road safety!)

1 Stop!

Don't be in a hurry to do things for him. He might surprise you with what he is able to do, so wait and see what he does.

2 Look!

Look at what your child does with the toys. It might not be what you think it should be! Let him use play to learn and explore. Remember there is no 'right' or 'wrong' way to do it. Try not to give him commands or instructions.

3 Listen!

Accept his ideas.

4 Think about what you are saying!

Remember that adults direct play through what they say as well as by what they do. Instead of telling your child what to do, try to…

- Comment on what he is doing, or about what is happening in the play.
  For example: *'That's the kettle – for making tea. You're putting water in now – I see. Lots of water. Oh look, it's full.'*

- Respond to what he says.
  For example: playing with dolls
  Child: *'Baby goes there. Baby in bed.'*
  Parent: *'Yes, baby is sleeping. She's tired.'*

- Repeat his idea back to him.
  For example: building with Lego®
  Child: *'That's where the driver sits.'*
  Parent: *'The driver sits there… I see.'*

- Add to his idea.
  For example: playing with farm set
  Child: *'There's the tractor.'*
  Parent: *'The farmer is driving the tractor. He's going into the field.'*

> To follow my child's lead I need to:
> - Stop
> - Look
> - Listen
> - Comment and respond
>
> Have a go at letting him take the lead in play!

'Keeping things simple' handout 1 of 2

Think

When I am playing with my child, what is the typical number of words in his sentences?

Why might it be helpful to think about the language I use when talking to my child and to match my language to my child's?

What do I need to 'do more of', or 'do differently', in order to match my language to my child?

Why we might be tempted to use more complicated words and sentences when talking to a child:

- We may think it encourages their language development
- Some children seem to have a natural interest in language and learning new words, and we want to encourage this
- We may be concerned they are behind with their talking.

Why might it be helpful for me to match my language to my child's?

- It encourages him to use words and sentences that he can manage comfortably
- It makes my language easier for him to understand
- A child who stammers may find it harder to be fluent when he is:
  - — trying to say a long, complicated sentence that is more difficult to organise in his mind
  - — trying to remember more complicated words that he is not sure of.

What do I need to 'do more of' or 'do differently' in order to match my language to my child's?

- Sit back and listen to how your child talks
- Notice the words that he usually uses. Try to use the same sorts of words as he does rather than teach him more difficult words. For example, say he is 'kind' rather than 'thoughtful'; refer to a 'glider' as a 'plane' rather than introduce the word 'glider'.
- How many words does he put together in a sentence? Try to keep your sentences about the same length as his, or slightly longer.
- Some children ask lots of questions and are keen to find out things. Think about how much detail you need to include in your answer. Generally, keep your explanations short and simple. For example, 'It's a plane that hasn't got an engine. It works by being blown by the wind'.
- Try to talk to your child about what is taking place in the 'here and now'. Keep to his topic of conversation and talk to him about what he is doing and what he is focused on.

Parents sometimes worry that using simpler language will affect the development of their child's talking, particularly when their child is already having some difficulty in saying some things correctly. Please do not worry. Asking parents to think about their talking in this way has been found to encourage rather than discourage language development.

If your child says a word incorrectly, or misses a word out, help him by modelling how it's done rather than 'correcting' him.

'Mummy, there's a tat'	*'Oh yes, there's a cat'*
'He catched the man'	*'He caught the man, did he?'*
'Dolly _ tired'	*'You're right, dolly is tired'*

When you model a word or sentence for your child in this way:

- Don't ask him to say it correctly after you
- Simply let him listen to you.

This is how children learn best.

- Listen
- Use the same words as child
- Use same sentence length as child
- Keep explanations short and simple
- Keep to 'here' and 'now'.

'Balancing comments and questions' handout

Think

When I am playing with my child, do I mainly make comments on what he is doing, or do I mainly ask him questions? Or do I already have a balance of comments and questions?

Here are some examples of comments and questions to help you decide:

'What colour is this car?'	Question
'Oh look, dolly's going to bed'	Comment
'That's a good idea, putting those animals in there'	Comment
'Where are you going to put that piece?'	Question
'You look as if you're having lots of fun'	Comment
'Why are you giving dolly a drink?'	Question

Why might it be helpful to have a balance of comments and questions when playing with my child?

What do I need to 'do more of', or 'do differently', in order to have a balance of comments and questions?

Adults often find it easier or more natural to ask questions than to make comments. They feel that by asking a question they are more likely to get a response.

We usually ask questions:

- To get some information
- To get a conversation going, particularly if a child is not saying very much
- As a way of suggesting what to do next
- To show how much a child knows
- To encourage a child to learn new things

Why might it be helpful to have a balance of comments and questions when playing with my child?

- Making comments on what a child is doing shows him that you are interested.
- When you ask a question, a child may feel he <u>has</u> to say something; he then needs to think of the answer and organise the sentence in the right way. Some children find this a bit of a challenge particularly while they are concentrating on playing.
- When you make comments your child can do things as quickly or slowly as he likes and he won't feel the need to rush to try to respond.
- Making comments on what a child is focused on will help develop his language as he hears you modelling different vocabulary and sentences to him. A child whose talking is delayed for his age may also find it easier to understand when comments involve the here and now.
- Comments can also get a conversation started and will give your child something to respond to.

What do I need to 'do more of' or 'do differently' in order to have a balance between comments and questions?

It is OK to ask questions, but before you ask a question, think to yourself…

- Do I need to ask this question? You may already know the answer and are just checking your child's knowledge.
- How complicated is this question to answer? Some questions involve a simple short answer, for example:
  'What's teddy doing?', *'Do you want a biscuit or a sweet?'*,
  whereas others involve a more complicated answer, for example:
  'What's going to happen if you put that marble there?'
- Will this question change the pace of play?
- How can I change this question into a comment? For example:
  'What's that?' becomes *'Look at that train'* or *'What's dolly doing?'* becomes *'Dolly's having a bath'*
  Sometimes we ask a question just with the ending. For example:
  'He's running, <u>isn't he</u>?' or *'You like dogs, <u>don't you</u>?'*
  All you need to do here is take off the ending and you will have changed the question into a comment.
- Remember to ask questions one at a time and give your child plenty of time to answer each question.
- It's OK not to speak, to allow the silence while people are thinking.

Five steps to making more comments

1 Look!

Look at what your child does with the toys. Try not to give him commands or instructions.

2 Comment on what he is doing, or about what is happening in the play.

For example:

'That's the kettle – for making tea. You're putting water in now – I see. Lots of water. Oh look, it's full.'

3 Respond to what he says.

For example: playing with dolls

Child: *'Baby goes there. Baby in bed'*

Parent: *'Yes, baby's sleeping. She's tired.'*

4 Repeat his idea back to him.

For example: building with Lego®

Child: *'That's where the driver sits'*

Parent: *'The driver sits there… I see.'*

5 Add to his idea.

For example: playing with farm set

Child: *'There's the tractor'*

Parent: *'The farmer is driving the tractor. He's going into the field.'*

'My rate of talking and use of pauses' handout

Think

When I am playing with my child, what speed or rate does he typically talk at?

____

Do I talk as slowly as my child or do I go faster?

____

Do I make use of pauses when I talk?

____

His speed: Slow / Moderate / Fast / Variable ______________________________

My speed: Same as his / Slower / Faster / Variable ______________________________

My pauses: Hardly ever / Sometimes / Often ______________________________

Why might it be helpful to think about my rate of talking and make use of pauses when talking to my child?

____

____

____

What do I need to 'do more of', or 'do differently' in order to talk a bit more slowly and make use of pauses?

____

____

____

You and your child do not necessarily speak any faster or slower than anyone else. However, a child who stammers usually finds it easier to be fluent when he speaks more slowly. Each child seems to have a different rate at which he is able to achieve fluency. You can help your child to take his time when talking by modelling a slower rate and using pauses, particularly if you naturally use a faster rate than your child does.

Why might it be helpful for me to talk more slowly and to make use of pauses?

- It gives the child more time to think and plan what he's trying to say.
- It gives him more time to organise what he would like to say when it's his turn.
- It makes your speech easier for him to understand.
- It gives him the feeling that there is plenty of time so he doesn't need to rush.
- It gives him time to go at his own pace.
- It encourages him to take his time, talk more slowly and use pauses.
- Generally, when a child talks more slowly it is easier for him to be more fluent.

What do I need to 'do more of' or 'do differently' in order to talk slowly and make use of pauses?

- Listen to how your child talks when he is relaxed and calm.
- Try to go at about the same rate or even a little more slowly.
- Try to pause before you say something as well as between sentences.
- You may find it helpful to tape-record yourself to listen to how slowly you are both speaking. You can then decide whether you need to make any changes.
- Even though you are talking slowly, try to keep it sounding interesting and as natural as possible. Try not to be 'choppy' or to speak like a robot.
- Remember that talking slowly or pausing more may feel rather strange to begin with - it takes practice.

Remember, although it may be tempting to ask your child to 'slow down', the best way to help him give himself more time when talking is for *you* to talk slowly and make use of pauses.

'Eye contact and talking' handout

Think

When my child is speaking, where is he looking?

How might developing my child's eye contact also help him to be more fluent?

Why do we need to look at people during a conversation?

- So that they will know we are talking to them.
- So that we can see if they are interested in what we are saying.
- So that we can see if they want to say something and we need to stop talking.
- So the speaker knows we are listening to them.

Why do we sometimes look away when we are speaking?

- To think about what we are saying.

What can happen if we look at something interesting while we are talking about something else?

- We can get distracted and forget what we are talking about.

Observe

Notice what people do when they are having a conversation.
When do they do most of the looking?

- When they are listening and sometimes when they are speaking.

When do they look away?

- When they are bored with listening.
- When they are thinking about what to say next.

Different types of looking:

1 normal looking
2 staring
3 looking away

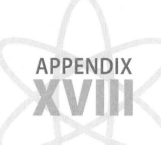

Looking and fluency

What could I do to help my child use more eye contact when he is talking?

- Make sure I'm looking at him.
- Touch him to get his attention.
- Say his name.
- Keep my eyes at the same level as his.
- Bring the object of his attention, such as a toy or a book, up to the level of my face.

A secret signal

You and your child could decide on a secret signal that you will use to remind him to look at you when he is speaking.

Questions for the SLT to ask in Palin PCI sessions

APPENDIX XIX

1 What have we/you found out about why your child stammers?
(When does he stammer more?)
(What seems to affect his fluency?)

2 What do you think he needs to do to be more fluent?

3 What are you already doing to help him to be more fluent?
(What do you do or say to help him when he is stammering?)

4 When are you doing that on the video?

Special Times task sheet: Scott

APPENDIX XX

Name of parent *Carly*
Name of child *Scott*
Number of Special Times *3*
Targets for Special Times *Watching and waiting*

DATE	ACTIVITY	COMMENTS ABOUT THE TARGETS
Tuesday	*Playing with Duplo*	*I liked watching and waiting while Scott was playing and talking – it was nice and relaxing, not having to think about what I should be doing or saying.*
Thursday	*Puzzle*	*Scott seems a lot calmer when I take a back seat – I think we both prefer it like this. I just let him sort out how to do the puzzle instead of taking over when it was difficult.*
Saturday	*Playing with train track*	*It was fun.*

IN ONE SENTENCE, WRITE DOWN WHAT YOU HAVE LEARNT FROM THIS WEEK'S ACTIVITIES

'Building my child's confidence' handout

Think

What is confidence?

What can I do to develop my child's confidence?

What has confidence got to do with stammering?

How to build my child's confidence

(Based on Faber & Mazlish, 1980)

1 Notice the good stuff!
Start to look out for something your child has done well or for something about his character you can praise. It doesn't have to be big – noticing the small things is a very good habit.

2 Comment on the good stuff
Show your child you have noticed by talking about it:

'I see you have put all your cars away.'

'You have coloured this in very well, keeping inside the lines and using lots of different colours.'

'I spy a clean plate – you have eaten all your food, every single bit.'

'When your sister fell over you helped her get up and looked after her.'

3 Give your child a positive label for it

This will help him store up a list of positive things about himself in his head, developing his self-image: 'My strong points…'

> *'I can see you have put all your cars away. You are very helpful.'*
>
> *'You have coloured this in very well. That was very careful and artistic of you.'*
>
> *'I spy a clean plate… You have been very sensible and helpful.'*
>
> *'When your sister… That was a very kind thing to do.'*

4 Watch out that you don't take the praise away again

It can be tempting to follow up praise with a sting in the tail! For example:

> *'Well done for putting your own socks on, that was really grown up of you. Why can't you do that every morning?'*

This is giving praise with one hand and taking it away with the other.

5 Make sure that your praise is sincere

If a child realises that you don't mean what you say, your praise is wasted, so try to keep it accurate and truthful.

6 Think about how you handle praise

What did you say when someone last praised you?

'I really like what you're wearing.'

'Oh, I just grabbed the first thing that came to hand.'

How did that make the praiser feel?

What could you have said instead?

Are you giving your child a good model for how to give and receive praise?

Building confidence

- Notice something good
- Describe what you have noticed
- Give the child a word or phrase to add to his list of 'My strong points'

'Openness about stammering' handout 1 of 2

APPENDIX XXII

Think

What do I do or say when I notice that my child is struggling to do something (eg, do up his buttons, colour in a picture, use a skipping rope)?

What do I do or say when my child is struggling to talk?

People used to think that if you drew a child's attention to his stammering, you would make it worse. There is no evidence for this. In fact, we now think the opposite:

Children may find it helpful to have their difficulty brought out into the open.

Some older children who stammer say they thought their stammer was something shameful that they had to hide from everybody. What gave them that idea?

Being open about your child's stammering may help him feel better about it, and this might stop him from feeling it is something he should try to hide from people.

Some things that other parents say

'Some words are really tricky to get out, aren't they?'

'That got a bit stuck, didn't it?'

'Well done, you got there in the end!'

Giving my child advice when he stammers

What do I sometimes say to my child when he stammers?

A natural reaction for parents is to give their child advice when he stammers, such as 'Slow down', 'Take a breath', etc. Such comments can be helpful to some children, but we typically advise parents to be careful about the amount of advice they give their child.

Why might giving advice not be very helpful for my child?

Is there something I could do with my own way of talking that might help him when he stammers?

Praise log

APPENDIX XXIII

What you praised	What you said Describe what it is you are praising, then add a praise word: 'That's very … of you.'	What your child did afterwards
Putting his toys away	I noticed that you've put all your toys in the toybox. That's so helpful.	He smiled and said 'I'm getting good at that now.'

With acknowledgement to: Faber, A. and Mazlish, E. (1980) *How to Talk So Kids will Listen and Listen So Kids will Talk.*

'Taking turns to talk' handout 1 of 2

Think

When my family is together:

Who does most of the talking? ____________________

Who does most of the listening? ____________________

Who does most of the interrupting? ____________________

What can happen when we don't take turns in conversations?

____

____

Why might it be helpful for my child who stammers if we all took turns?

____

____

Often, in families:

- Everybody talks at once
- People interrupt one another
- No one listens
- One person does all the talking
- People are afraid of interrupting the stammering child.

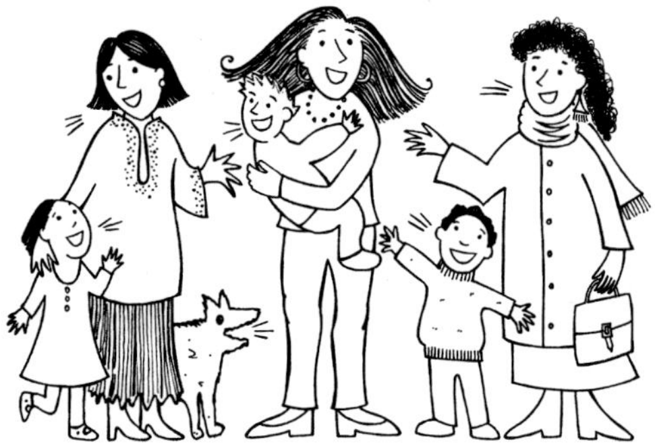

Typical group behaviour!

When this happens:

- People are not *taking turns*
- Everyone is competing for time to talk.

It is especially likely if you have a large family where everyone has something to say!

Why would it be helpful to make sure everyone has a turn (including the child who stammers)?

Competing for a turn to talk might make things difficult for the child who stammers:

- He feels that he must speak quickly in order to get a turn
- He has less time to think of what he wants to say
- He has to cope with people interrupting him
- He may try to interrupt others
- It is harder for him to be calm and take his time
- Once he gets his turn he may not want to give it up! So he may talk for too long and not let others have a turn speaking.

What are the rules for good turn-taking?

- When one person is speaking, others listen
- No one interrupts
- Everybody has a turn
- Vary who gets to speak first
- No one should speak for too long.

How can I improve my turn-taking?

- Watch! Listen! Wait! to ensure that your child has finished speaking before you start to talk
- Count to two in your head before responding to your child's speech
- When your child speaks to you, respond either verbally or non-verbally (eg, smiling, nodding).

How can I encourage other members of the family to take turns?

- Teach everybody in your family the rules of turn-taking:
  - Play games where you have to take turns, for example Snakes and Ladders; Ludo; Snap; Monopoly; building something as a team.
  - Play the Microphone Game.

The Microphone Game

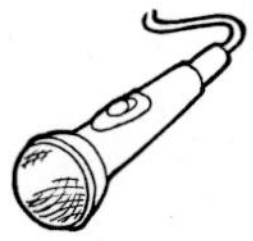

- Choose something that will be the microphone, eg, a pencil, a wooden spoon
- Put the microphone in the middle
- When somebody wants to talk, they pick up the microphone
- Nobody else can talk or interrupt; they are listening
- When the speaker has finished, the microphone is put down
- The next speaker picks up the microphone and takes a turn to talk
- Everybody has a chance to speak
- Nobody should take all the turns
- Nobody should take very long turns.

You can play the Microphone Game at mealtimes or even in the car (except for the driver!).

'Helping my child to deal with his feelings' handout

FEELINGS AND HOW WE HANDLE THEM			
Feeling	What kinds of things make my child feel this way?	How does he show this feeling?	What do I normally do or say when he feels like this?
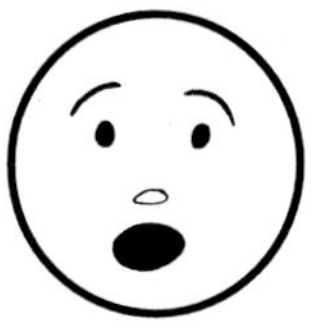 Fear			
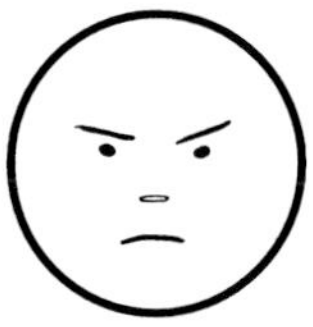 Anger			
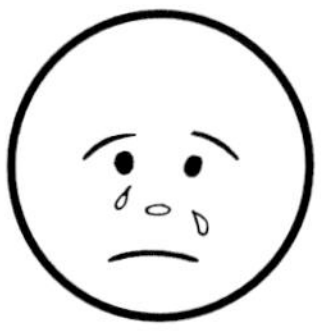 Sadness			
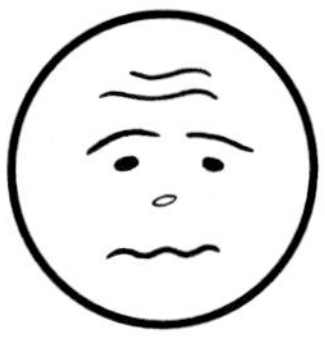 Worry			

How we sometimes react

If you are very worried about something, and someone tells you:

'Cheer up! Don't worry! It might never happen,'

does that make you feel better?

APPENDIX XXV Helping my child to deal with feelings

People often think that, instead of listening to how you feel and showing sympathy, they should tell you to stop feeling that way. But does that make the feeling go away? Sometimes it can make it worse.

It might be more helpful if they said:

'You poor thing. You are really worried about that, aren't you'?

Parents may do the same with children:

The child says	***The parent says***
I hate my brother.	*No you don't, you like him really.*
I'm worried nobody will play with me at preschool.	*Don't worry. Of course they will.*
I'm scared of the dark.	*Don't be silly. There's nothing to be frightened of.*

The parent is telling the child he does not feel like that.

But does that make the child feel better?

Is the child likely to keep telling his parents how he feels, or will he learn to keep his feelings to himself?

A different way of reacting

The child says	***The parent says***
I hate my brother.	*You sound pretty cross with him. He must have done something big to upset you this much.*
I'm worried nobody will play with me at preschool.	*I can see that you are really anxious about being on your own, aren't you?*
I'm scared of the dark.	*You seem very frightened about having the light off.*

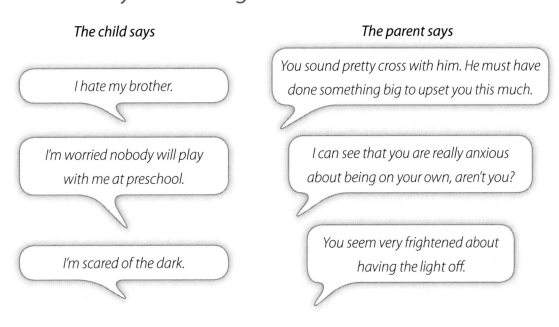

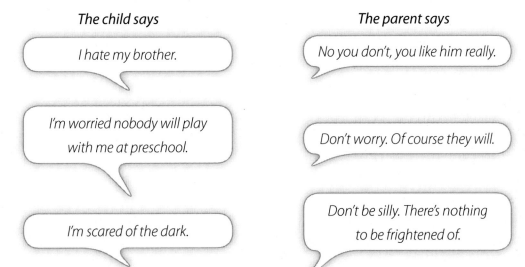

APPENDIX XXV Helping my child to deal with feelings

This time the parent is listening to what the child says, and accepting that he feels that way.

He is showing he has listened and he believes the child by describing the feelings back to him.

When a child can't put it into words

Sometimes a child is unable to tell you how he feels, but you can see something is wrong. He may need your help putting it into words:

- 'That's an unhappy face' 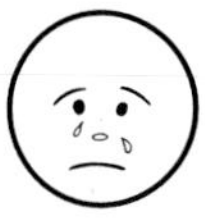
- 'You look very cross to me' 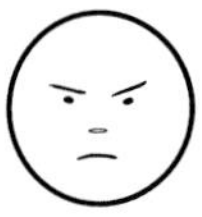
- 'You seem really worried' 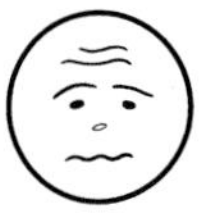

Not only are you showing that you have noticed how he feels, you are giving him the words to describe the emotion.

Encouraging the child to show his feelings

Listening carefully and then describing the child's feelings will let him know it's OK to show how he feels.

You could also encourage him to vent his feelings more:

- 'It's OK, have a good cry'
- 'Why don't you hit that pillow as hard as you can to show me how cross you are?'
- 'Shall we write down all the things you are worried about?'

Based on model suggested by Faber and Mazlish (1980)

'The child whose standards are too high' handout 1 of 2

Think

What kinds of things does my child want to get exactly right or do well in?

How does he react when it's not quite right or he's not the winner?

How might this have something to do with his stammering?

A vicious circle

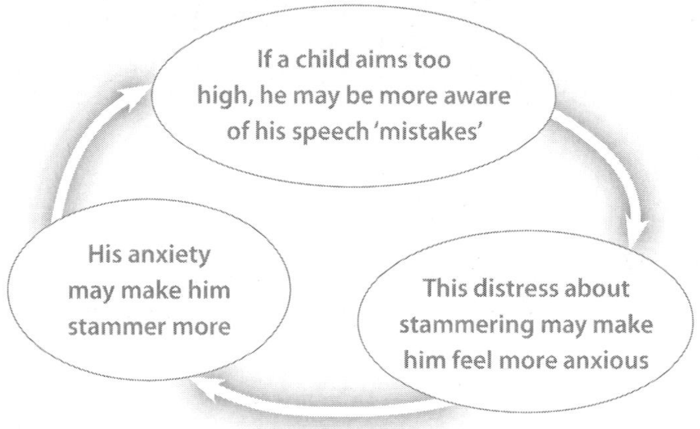
If a child aims too high, he may be more aware of his speech 'mistakes'
This distress about stammering may make him feel more anxious
His anxiety may make him stammer more

How can parents help?

Think

How do I react when I make a mistake or things go wrong for me?

For example:

- When I lose my keys
- When I forget something
- When I make a mistake.

When something goes wrong for us, we often show anger or distress.
If we make a big deal of it, the child will think it is a big deal.
If we are able to make light of it, the child will see that things are not so bad after all when we make mistakes.

How could I react so that I show my child that I feel OK about getting something wrong?

I could try ....

....

....

Think

How do I react when my child gets something wrong?

....

....

....

How could I react so that my child feels OK about not getting it quite right?

....

....

....

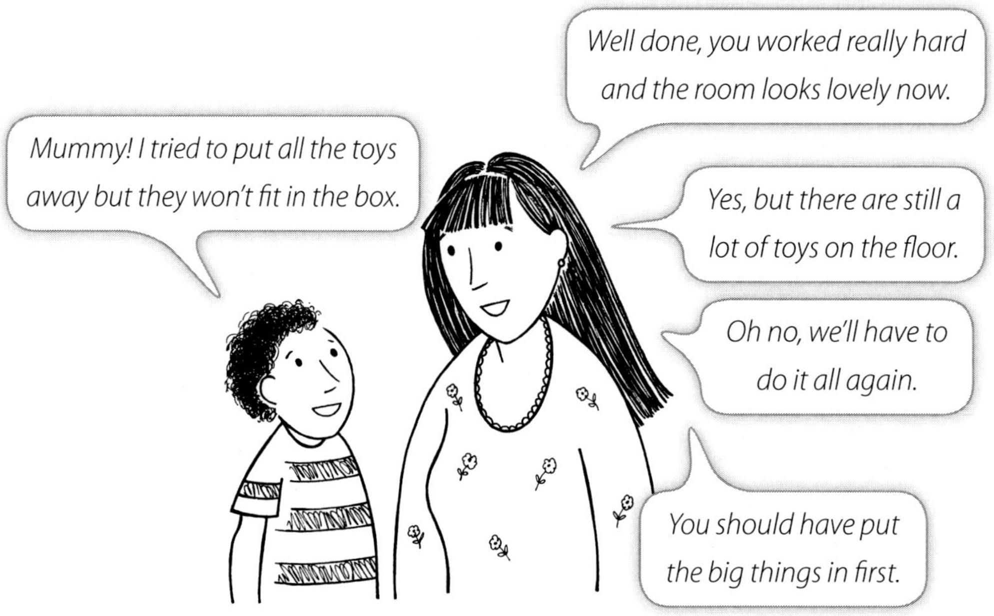
Mummy! I tried to put all the toys away but they won't fit in the box.
Well done, you worked really hard and the room looks lovely now.
Yes, but there are still a lot of toys on the floor.
Oh no, we'll have to do it all again.
You should have put the big things in first.

'Managing my child's behaviour' handout 1 of 3

Think

When my child misbehaves, do I ever react differently because of his stammering? ______

Why? ______

An example of when I have reacted differently when he did something wrong ______

How would I have reacted if his brother or sister had done the same thing wrong? ______

Brothers or sisters of children who stammer might think it's not fair if a different set of rules apply to them!

What could happen if I keep on treating him differently because of his stammer? ______

Some older children who stammer say that they can get away with things because their parents or teachers are worried about telling them off!

A child who stammers may be told off for interrupting when he is speaking well, but allowed to interrupt when he is stammering. What kind of message is he getting? ______

Challenging behaviours

I find it difficult to know how to handle my child when he ______

How to react when a child won't co-operate

Example: You put your child to bed but he keeps coming downstairs
Possible reaction:

- ***Tell him off***
- ***Shout at him***
- ***Ignore him***
- ***Give in and let him watch TV with you***
- ***Threaten him***
- ***Take him back up and get into bed with him***
- ***Smack him***

Some different ways to react:

- Describe the problem: 'I see someone has come downstairs who is supposed to be in bed.'
- Give information: 'Children who don't stay in bed don't get enough sleep and they get tired and grumpy.'
- Say it with a word: 'Bed!'
- Talk about your feelings: 'I feel disappointed that you are down here and I'm worried about how tired you will be tomorrow.'
- Write a note: 'Go back to bed.'

Thinking of different ways to handle a problem

We often get stuck when we are faced with a problem. We think we have tried everything and nothing works.

Sometimes we need help in thinking of some new ideas for tackling it. But who can we ask?

Ask your children to help you!

Children can be very creative thinkers.

How to solve a problem ______________________

____

____

1 Write the problem down
'My problem is ______________________'

2 Brainstorm ideas
Take it in turns to think of different ideas to handle the problem. Don't judge the ideas. Write each one down, even if you don't like the sound of it or you have tried it before. Encourage wacky ideas – you never know! Keep on thinking up new ideas until there are no more.

3 Think about each idea

Decide whether you want to give it a try, then keep it in or cross it out.

4 Put the ideas in order

Choose the idea you would like to try first, then second, etc.

5 Try it out!

Making a child feel good when he gets it right

> ***Why do teachers give out stars or merits?***
> ***Why do bosses give employees a bonus?***
> ***How do people train dogs to do tricks?***

Merits, treats, bonuses, stars, house points: these are all used to reward something good and encourage us to do more of the same.

Sometimes it helps children to change their behaviour if there is an extra reward. Star charts can be helpful.

- Decide with your child what the target will be

  For example: *'When I go to bed I will stay there.'*

- Make a star chart with your child
- Tell your child that each day he goes to bed and stays there, he will be given a star to stick on his star chart
- You may decide to tell your child that if he gets five stars he will get a special treat, like a trip to the park
- Beware of making the treat too exciting or expensive, you might not be able to follow it next time!
- Some children don't need the extra treat – the star is rewarding enough.

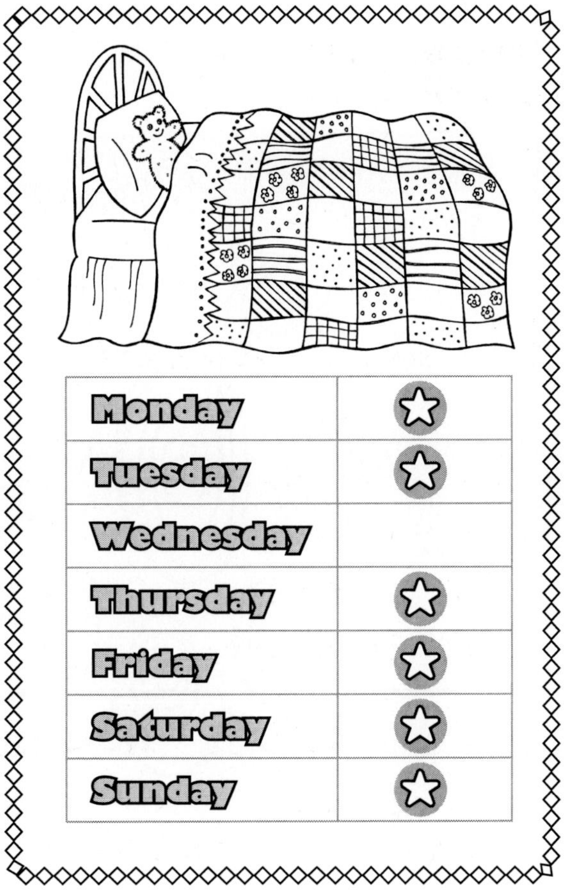
Monday
Tuesday
Wednesday
Thursday
Friday
Saturday
Sunday

Tortoise Talking practice chart

Tortoise Talking

Tick the box when you have practised

☐	☐	☐	☐	☐
☐	☐	☐	☐	☐
☐	☐	☐	☐	☐

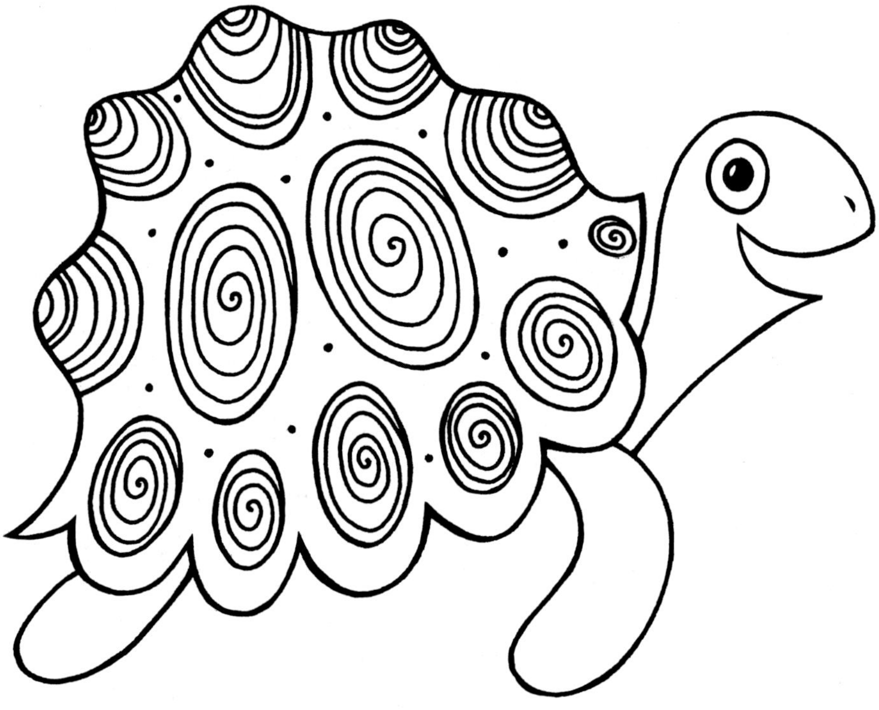

Bus Talking practice chart

APPENDIX XXIX

Bus Talking

Put a sticker or a stamp every time you do a practice or when you just do Bus Talking

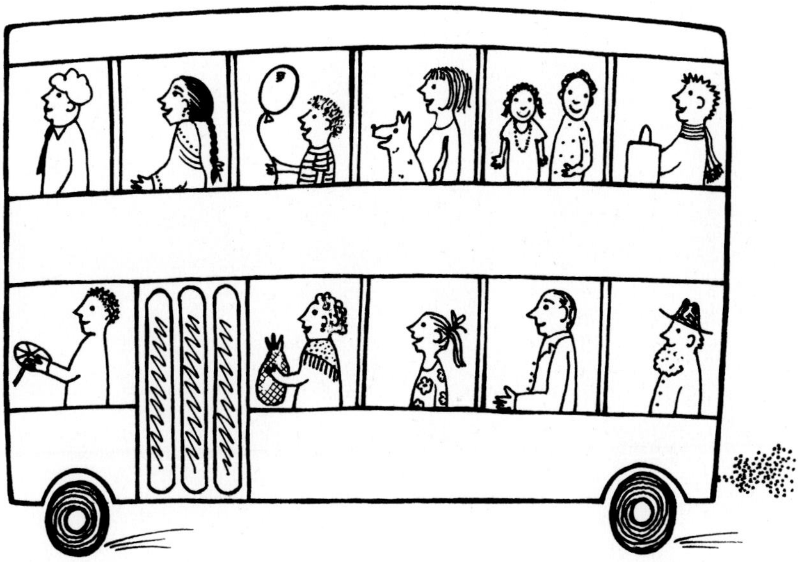

Palin PCI home programme record

APPENDIX XXX

What helps?

What seems to help my child to be more fluent?

When he ______________________________

____

____

When I ______________________________

____

____

Special Times

I will do ______ Special Times each week.

My first Special Time target will be ______________________________

____

____

My second Special Time target will be ______________________________

____

____

My third Special Time target will be ______________________________

____

____

Family strategies

My family strategies:

1 Building my child's confidence

2 ______________________________

3 ______________________________

☏ SLT telephone number ______________________________

☏ Day and time I will telephone ______________________________

Resources

Further reading

- De'Ath E & Slater D (eds), 1992, *Parenting Threads: Caring for Children when Couples Part*, Stepfamily Publications, London.
- Dyregrov A, 1990, *Grief in Children: A Handbook for Adults*, Jessica Kingsley Publishers, London.
- Van den Berg M, 1994, *The Three Birds*, Magination Press, New York.
- Sunderland M, 2003, *The Day the Sea Went Out and Never Came Back*, Speechmark Publishing, Milton Keynes.
- Kerr J, 2002, *Goodbye Mog*, Collins, London.

Useful addresses

UK

- The Michael Palin Centre for Stammering Children
  website: www.stammeringcentre.org
  email: info@stammeringcentre.org
- The British Stammering Association
  website: www.stammering.org
  email: mail@stammering.org
- Royal College of Speech and Language Therapists
  website: www.rcslt.org
  email: postmaster@rcslt.org

USA

- The Stuttering Foundation
  website: www.stutteringhelp.org
- National Stuttering Association
  website: www.nsastutter.org
- Stuttering homepage
  website: www.stutteringhomepage.org

Europe

- European League of Stuttering Associations
  website: www.stuttering.ws

Australia

- Australian Speak Easy Association
  website: www.speakeasy.org.au

South Africa

- Speak Easy South Africa
  website: www.speakeasy.org.za

International

- International Stuttering Association
  website: www.stutterisa.org

References

Adams AR, 1990, 'The Demands and Capacities Model 1: Theoretical Elaborations', *Journal of Fluency Disorders* 15, pp135–141.

Allen JL & Rapee RM, 2005, 'Anxiety Disorders', Graham P (ed), *Cognitive Behaviour Therapy for Children and Families*, pp300–319, Cambridge University Press, Cambridge.

Ambrose NG & Yairi E, 1994, 'The Development of Awareness of Stuttering in Preschool Children', *Journal of Fluency Disorders* 19, pp229–245.

Ambrose NG & Yairi E, 1999, 'Normative Disfluency Data for Early Childhood Stuttering', *Journal of Speech, Language and Hearing Research* 42, pp895–909.

Anderson JD & Conture EG, 2000, 'Language Abilities of Children who Stutter: A Preliminary Study', *Journal of Fluency Disorders* 25, pp283–304.

Anderson JD, Pellowski MW & Conture EG, 2005, 'Childhood Stuttering and Dissociations across Linguistic Domains', *Journal of Fluency Disorders* 30, pp219–253.

Anderson JD, Pellowski MW, Conture E & Kelly E, 2003, 'Temperamental Characteristics of Young Children who Stutter', *Journal of Speech, Language and Hearing Research* 46, pp1221–1233.

Andrews C, Hoddinott S, Craig A, Howie P, Feyer AM & Neilson M, 1983, 'Stuttering: A Review of Research and Findings and Theories Circa 1982', *Journal of Speech and Hearing Disorders* 48, pp226–246.

Andronico M & Blake I, 1971, 'The Application of Filial Therapy to Young Children with Stuttering Problems', *Journal of Speech and Hearing Disorders* 36, pp377–381.

Au-Yeung J, Howell P, Davis S, Charles N & Sackin S, 2000, 'UCL Survey on Bilingualism and Stuttering', Bosshardt HG, Yaruss JS & Peters HFM (eds), *Fluency Disorders: Theory, Research, Treatment and Self-help. Proceedings of the Third World Congress on Fluency Disorders*, University of Nijmegen Press, Nyborg, Denmark.

Beck JS, 1995, *Cognitive Therapy: Basics and Beyond*, Guilford Press, New York, NY.

Bernstein Ratner N, 1992, 'Measurable Outcomes of Instruction to Modify Normal Parent-Child Verbal Interactions: Implications for Indirect Stuttering Therapy', *Journal of Speech and Hearing Disorders* 35, pp14–20.

Bernstein Ratner N, 1995, 'Treating the Child who Stutters with Concomitant Language or Phonological Impairment', *Language, Speech and Hearing Services in Schools* 26, pp180–186.

Bernstein Ratner N, 1997a, 'Stuttering: A Psycholinguistic Perspective', Curlee R & Siegel GM (eds), *Nature and Treatment of Stuttering: New Directions*, Allyn & Bacon, Boston, MA.

Bernstein Ratner N, 1997b, 'Linguistic Behaviors at the Onset of Stuttering', Hulstijn W, Peters HF & van Lieshout PH (eds), *Motor Control, Brain Research and Fluency Disorders*, Elsevier, Amsterdam.

Bernstein Ratner N, 2001, 'What Child Language Research Contributes to Understanding and Treating Stuttering', Paper presented at the annual convention of American Speech-Language-Hearing Association Conference, New Orleans, November, 2001.

Bernstein Ratner N & Sih CC, 1987, 'Effects of Gradual Increases in Sentence Length and Complexity on Children's Dysfluency', *Journal of Speech and Hearing Disorders* 52, pp278-287.

Biggart A, Cook FM & Fry J, 2007, 'The Role of Parents in Stuttering Treatment from a Cognitive Behavioural Perspective', *Proceedings of The Fifth World Congress on Fluency Disorders, Dublin, Ireland, 25–28th July, 2006*, pp268–375.

Bishop JH, Williams HG & Cooper WA, 1991, 'Age and Task Complexity Variables in Motor Performance of Children with Articulation-disordered Stuttering, and Normal Speech', *Journal of Fluency Disorders* 16, pp219–228.

Blood GW, Ridenour VJ, Qualls CD & Hammer CS, 2003, 'Co-occurring Disorders in Children who Stutter', *Journal of Communication Disorders* 36, pp427–448.

Bloodstein O, 1995, *A Handbook on Stuttering*, Singular Publishing Group, San Diego, CA.

Bloodstein O & Bernstein Ratner N, 2007, *A Handbook on Stuttering*, Thomson/Cengage, Clifton Park, NY.

Bonelli P, Dixon M, Bernstein Ratner N & Onslow M, 2000, 'Child and Parent Speech and Language Following the Lidcombe Program of Early Stuttering Intervention', *Clinical Linguistics and Phonetics* 14, pp427–446.

Botterill W, Kelman E & Rustin L, 1991, 'Parents and their Pre-school Stuttering Child', Rustin L (ed), *Parents, Families and the Stuttering Child*, Far Communications Ltd, Kibworth.

Braun AR, Varga M, Stager S, Schulz G, Selbie S, Maisog JM, Carson RE & Ludlow CL, 1997, 'Altered Patterns of Cerebral Activity During Speech and Language Production in Developmental Stuttering. An H2(15)O Positron Emission Tomography Study', *Brain* 120 (Pt 5), pp761–784.

Byrd K & Cooper EB, 1989, 'Expressive and Receptive Language Skills in Stuttering Children', *Journal of Fluency Disorders* 14, pp121–126.

Caruso AJ, Max L & McClowry TM, 1999, 'Perspectives on Stuttering as a Motor Speech Disorder', Caruso AJ & Strand EA (eds), *Clinical Management of Motor Speech Disorders in Children,* Thieme, New York, NY.

Conti-Ramsden G, Hutcheson GD & Grove J, 1995, 'Contingency and Breakdown: Children with SLI and their Conversations with Mothers and Fathers', *Journal of Speech and Hearing Research* 38, pp1290–1302.

Conture EG, 1990, *Stuttering*, Prentice-Hall, Englewood Cliffs, NJ.

Conture E, 2001, *Stuttering: Its Nature, Diagnosis and Treatment*, Allyn & Bacon, Boston, MA.

Conture EG & Melnick KS, 1999, 'Parent-child Group Approach to Stuttering in Preschool Children', Onslow M & Packman A (eds), *The Handbook of Early Stuttering Intervention,* The Singular Publishing Group, London.

Conture E, Louko LJ & Edwards M, 1993, 'Simultaneously Treating Stuttering and Disordered Phonology in Children: Experimental Therapy, Preliminary Findings', *American Journal of Speech-Language Pathology* 2, pp72–81.

Conture EG, Rothenberg M & Molitor RD, 1986, 'Electroglottographic Observations of Young Stutterers' Fluency', *Journal of Speech and Hearing Research* 29, pp384–393.

Cox N, Cook E, Ambrose N, Yairi E, Rydmarker S & Lundstrom C, 2000, 'The Illinois-Sweden-Israel Genetics of Stuttering Project', Paper presented at the Third World Congress on Fluency Disorders, Nyborg, Denmark.

Crichton-Smith I, 2002, 'Changing Conversational Dynamics: A Case Study in Parent-Child Interaction Therapy', *Proceedings of The Sixth Oxford Dysfluency Conference,* KLB Publications, Leicester.

Crichton-Smith I, Wright J & Stackhouse J, 2003, 'Attitudes of Speech and Language Therapists Towards Stammering: 1985 and 2000', *International Journal of Language and Communication Disorders* 38, pp213–234.

Cummins K & Hulme S, 1997, 'Video – A Reflective Tool', *Speech and Language Therapy in Practice*, pp 4–7.

Curlee R, 1999, *Stuttering and Related Disorders of Fluency*, Thieme Medical Publishers, New York, NY.

De Nil LF, Kroll RM, Kapur S & Houle S, 2000, 'A Positron Emission Tomography Study of Silent and Oral Single Word Reading in Stuttering and Nonstuttering Adults', *Journal of Speech, Language and Hearing Research* 43, pp1038–1053.

De Nil LF, Kroll RM, Lafaille SJ & Houle S, 2003, 'A Positron Emission Tomography Study of Short- and Long-term Treatment Effects on Functional Brain Activation in Adults who Stutter', *Journal of Fluency Disorders* 28, pp357–380.

De Shazer S, 1988, *Clues: Investigating Solutions in Brief Therapy*, Norton, New York, NY.

De Shazer, **S**, 1996, *Words Were Originally Magic*, Norton, New York, NY.

Douglas J, 2005, 'Behavioural Approaches to Eating and Sleeping Problems in Young Children', Graham P (ed), *Cognitive Behaviour Therapy for Children and Families,* Cambridge University Press, Cambridge.

Drayna DT, 1997, 'Genetic Linkage Studies of Stuttering: Ready for Prime Time?' *Journal of Fluency Disorders* 22, pp237–241.

Edwards S, Fletcher P, Garman M, Hughes A, Letts C & Sinka I, 1997, *The Reynell Developmental Language Scales III: The University of Reading Edition*, NFER-Nelson, Windsor.

Embrechts M & Ebben H, 1999, 'A Comparison between the Interactions of Stuttering and Nonstuttering Children and their Parents', Baker KL, Rustin L & Cook F (eds), *The Fifth Oxford Dysfluency Conference*, Kevin L Baker, Oxford.

Embrechts M, Ebben H, Franke P & van de Poel C, 2000, 'Temperament: A Comparison between Children who Stutter and Children who do not Stutter', Bosshardt HG, Yaruss JS & Peters HFM (eds), *Fluency Disorders: Theory, Research, Treatment and Self-help. Proceedings of the Third World Congress on Fluency Disorders,* University of Nijmegen Press, Nyborg, Denmark.

Epstein NB & Bishop DS, 1981, 'Problem-centered Systems Therapy of the Family', Gurman AS & Kniskern DP (eds), *Handbook of Family Therapy*, Brunner/Mazel, New York, NY.

Ezrati-Vinacour R, Platzky R & Yairi E, 2001, 'The Young Child's Awareness of Stuttering-like Disfluency', *Journal of Speech, Language and Hearing Research* 44, pp368–380.

Faber A & Mazlish E, 1980, *How to Talk so Kids will Listen and Listen so Kids will Talk*, Avon Books, New York, NY.

Farber S, 1981, *Identical Twins Reared Apart: A Reanalysis*, Basic Books, New York, NY.

Felsenfeld S, 1997, 'Epidemiology and Genetics of Stuttering', Curlee R & Siegel GM (eds), *Nature and Treatment of Stuttering: New Directions*, pp3–22, Allyn & Bacon, Boston, MA.

Foundas AL, Bollich AM, Corey DM, Hurley M & Heilman KM, 2001, 'Anomalous Anatomy of Speech and Language Areas in Adults with Persistent Developmental Stuttering', *Neurology* 57, pp207–215.

Fowlie GM & Cooper EB, 1978, 'Traits Attributed to Stuttering and Non-stuttering Children by their Mothers', *Journal of Fluency Disorders* 3, pp233–246.

Fox PT, Ingham RJ, Ingham JC, Hirsch TB, Downs JH, Martin C, Jerabek P, Glass T & Lancaster JL, 1996, 'A PET Study of the Neural Systems of Stuttering', *Nature* 382, pp158–161.

Fox PT, Ingham RJ, Ingham JC, Zamarripa F, Xiong JH & Lancaster JL, 2000, 'Brain Correlates of Stuttering and Syllable Production. A PET Performance-correlation Analysis', *Brain* 123 (Pt 10), pp1985–2004.

Franken MC, Kielstra-Van der Schalk CJ & Boelens H, 2005, 'Experimental Treatment of Early Stuttering: A Preliminary Study', *Journal of Fluency Disorders* 30, pp189-199.

Fransella F, 1972, *Personal Change and Reconstruction*, Academic Press, London.

Gaines ND, Runyan CM & Meyers SC, 1991, 'A Comparison of Young Stutterers' Fluent versus Stuttered Utterances on Measures of Length and Complexity', *Journal of Speech and Hearing Research* 34, pp37–42.

Girolametto L, Greenberg J & Manolson A, 1986, 'Developing Dialogue Skills: The Hanen Early Language Parent Program', *Seminars in Speech and Language* 7, pp367–382.

Girolametto L, Weitzman E, van Lieshout R & Duff D, 2000, 'Directiveness in Teachers' Language Input to Toddlers and Preschoolers in Day Care', *Journal of Speech, Language and Hearing Research* 43, pp1101–1114.

Girolametto L, Weitzman E, Wiigs M & Steig Pearce P, 1999, 'The Relationship between Maternal Language Measures and Language Development in Toddlers with Expressive Vocabulary Delay', *American Journal of Speech-Language Pathology* 8, pp364–374.

Gottwald SR & Starkweather CW, 1995, 'Fluency Intervention for Preschoolers and their Families in the Public Schools', *Language, Speech, and Hearing Services in Schools* 26, pp117–126.

Gottwald S & Starkweather C, 1999, 'Stuttering Prevention and Early Intervention: A Multiprocess Approach', Onslow M & Packman A (eds), *The Handbook of Early Stuttering Intervention,* Singular Publishing Group Inc, San Diego, CA.

Guitar B, 1998, *Stuttering: An Integrated Approach to its Nature and Treatment*, Williams & Wilkins, Baltimore, MD.

Guitar B, 2006, *Stuttering: An Integrated Approach to Its Nature and Treatment*, Lippincott Williams & Wilkins, Philadelphia, PA.

Guitar B & Marchinkoski L, 2001, 'Influence of Mothers' Slower Speech on their Children's Speech Rate', *Journal of Speech, Language and Hearing Research* 44, pp853–861.

Guitar B, Kopf-Schaefer HK, Donahue-Kilburg G & Bond L, 1992, 'Parental Verbal Interactions and Speech Rate: A Case Study in Stuttering', *Journal of Speech and Hearing Research* 35, pp742–754.

Hage A, 2000, 'Is There a Link between the Development of Cognitive-Linguistic Abilities in Children and the Course of Stuttering?', Bosshardt HG, Yaruss JS & Peters HFM (eds), *Fluency Disorders: Theory, Research, Treatment and Self-help. Proceedings of the Third World Congress on Fluency Disorders,* University of Nijmegen Press, Nyborg, Denmark.

Healey EC & Reid R, 2003, 'ADHD and Stuttering: A Tutorial', *Journal of Fluency Disorders* 28, pp79–93.

Healey EC, Reid R & Donaher J, 2005, 'Treatment of the Child who Stutters with Co-existing Learning, Behavioral, and Cognitive Challenges', Lees R & Stark C (eds), *The Treatment of Stuttering in the Young School-Aged Child,* Whurr Publishers, London.

Henderlong J & Lepper MR, 2002, 'The Effects of Praise on Children's Intrinsic Motivation: A Review and Synthesis', *Psychological Bulletin* 128, pp774–795.

Howell P & Au-Yeung J, 1995, 'Syntactic Determinants of Stuttering in the Spontaneous Speech of Normally Fluent and Stuttering Children', *Journal of Fluency Disorders* 20, pp317–330.

Howell P, Au-Yeung J & Sackin S, 1999, 'Exchange of Stuttering from Function Words to Content Words with Age', *Journal of Speech, Language and Hearing Research* 42, pp345–354.

Howell P, Davis S & Au-Yeung J, 2003, 'Syntactic Development in Fluent Children, Children who Stutter, and Children who have English as an Additional Language', *Child Language Teaching and Therapy* 19, pp311–337.

Howie PM, 1981, 'Concordance for Stuttering in Monozygotic and Dizygotic Twin Pairs', *Journal of Speech and Hearing Research* 24, pp317–321.

Hulme S, 2005, 'ACT! Innovative Training for Childcare Staff', *Bulletin*, pp12–13.

Ingham JC & Riley G, 1998, 'Guidelines for Documentation of Treatment Efficacy for Young Children who Stutter', *Journal of Speech, Language and Hearing Research* 41, pp753–770.

Irwin A, 1988, *Stammering in Young Children: A Practical Self-help Programme for Parents*, Thorsons Publishing Group, Wellingborough.

Jennische M & Sedin G, 1999, 'Speech and Language Skills in Children who Required Neonatal Intensive Care: Evaluation at 6.5 Years of Age Based on Interviews with Parents', *Acta Paediatrica* 88, pp975–982.

Johannsen HS, 2000, 'Design of the Longitudinal Study and Influence of Symptomatology: Heredity, Sex Ratio and Lateral Dominance on the Further Development of Stuttering', Bosshardt HG, Yaruss JS & Peters HFM (eds), *Fluency Disorders: Theory, Research, Treatment and Self-help. Proceedings of the Third World Congress on Fluency Disorders,* University of Nijmegen Press, Nyborg, Denmark.

Johnson W, 1942, 'A Study of the Onset and Development of Stuttering', *Journal of Speech Disorders* 7, pp251–257.

Jones M, Gebski V, Onslow M & Packman A, 2001, 'Design of Randomized Controlled Trials. Principles and Methods Applied to a Treatment for Early Stuttering', *Journal of Fluency Disorders* 26, pp247–267.

Jones M, Onslow M, Packman A, Williams S, Ormond T, Schwarz T & Gebski V, 2005, 'A Randomised Controlled Trial of the Lidcombe Program for Early Stuttering Intervention', *British Medical Journal* 331, pp659–661.

Kadi Hanifi K & Howell P, 1992, 'Syntactic Analysis of the Spontaneous Speech of Normally Fluent and Stuttering Children', *Journal of Fluency Disorders* 17, pp151–170.

Karrass J, Walden TA, Conture EG, Graham CG, Arnold HS, Hartfield KN & Schwenk KA, 2006, 'Relation of Emotional Reactivity and Regulation to Childhood Stuttering', *Journal of Communication Disorders* 39, pp402–423.

Kasprisin Burrelli A, Egolf DB & Shames GH, 1972, 'A Comparison of Parental Verbal Behavior with Stuttering and Nonstuttering Children', *Journal of Communication Disorders* 5, pp335–346.

Kelly E, 1994a, 'Mothers, Fathers, and their Children who Stutter: Paralinguistic Behaviors', Starkweather CW & Peters HFM (eds), *Stuttering: Proceedings of the First World Congress on Fluency Disorders,* University of Nijmegen Press, Nyborg, Denmark.

Kelly EM, 1994b, 'Speech Rates and Turn-taking Behaviors of Children who Stutter and their Fathers', *Journal of Speech and Hearing Research* 37, pp1284–1294.

Kelly EM, 1995, 'Parents as Partners: Including Mothers and Fathers in the Treatment of Children who Stutter', *Journal of Communication Disorders* 28, pp93–105.

Kelly EM & Conture EG, 1992, 'Speaking Rates, Response Time Latencies, and Interrupting Behaviors of Young Stutterers, Nonstutterers, and their Mothers', *Journal of Speech and Hearing Research* 35, pp1256–1267.

Kelly EM, Smith A & Goffman L, 1995, 'Orofacial Muscle Activity of Children who Stutter: A Preliminary Study', *Journal of Speech and Hearing Research* 38, pp1025–1036.

Kelly GA, 1955, *The Psychology of Personal Constructs: Clinical Diagnosis and Psychotherapy*, WW Norton & Co, New York, NY.

Kelman E & Schneider C, 1994, 'Parent-child Interaction: An Alternative Approach to the Management of Children's Language Difficulties', *Child Language Teaching and Therapy* 10, pp81–96.

Kidd KK, Kidd JR & Records MA, 1978, 'The Possible Causes of the Sex Ratio in Stuttering and its Implications', *Journal of Fluency Disorders* 3, pp13–23.

Kloth SAM, Janssen P, Kraaimaat FW & Brutten GJ, 1995a, 'Speech-Motor and Linguistic Skills of Young Stutterers Prior to Onset', *Journal of Fluency Disorders* 20, pp157–170.

Kloth SAM, Janssen P, Kraaimaat FW & Brutten GJ, 1995b, 'Communicative Behavior of Mothers of Stuttering and Nonstuttering High-risk Children prior to the Onset of Stuttering', *Journal of Fluency Disorders* 20, pp365–377.

Kloth SAM, Janssen P, Kraaimaat F & Brutten GJ, 1998, 'Child and Mother Variables in the Development of Stuttering among High-risk Children: A Longitudinal Study', *Journal of Fluency Disorders* 23, pp217–230.

Kloth SAM, Kraaimaat FW, Janssen P & Brutten GJ, 1999, 'Persistence and Remission of Incipient Stuttering among High-risk Children', *Journal of Fluency Disorders* 24, pp253–256.

Kully D & Langevin M, 2005, 'Evidence-based Practice in Fluency Disorders', *ASHA Leader* 10, pp10–11, 23.

Langlois A, Hanrahan LL & Inouye LL, 1986, 'A Comparison of Interactions between Stuttering Children, Nonstuttering Children, and their Mothers', *Journal of Fluency Disorders* 11, pp263–273.

LDA, 1988, '*What's Wrong? Cards*', Living and Learning, Cambridge.

Lincoln MA & Onslow M, 1997, 'Long-term Outcome of Early Intervention for Stuttering', *American Journal of Speech-Language Pathology* 6, pp51–58.

Logan K & Conture E, 1995, 'Length, Grammatical Complexity and Rate Differences in Stuttered and Fluent Conversational Utterances of Children who Stutter', *Journal of Fluency Disorders* 20, pp35–61.

Logan KJ & Conture EG, 1997, 'Selected Temporal, Grammatical, and Phonological Characteristics of Conversational Utterances produced by Children who Stutter', *Journal of Speech, Language and Hearing Research* 40, pp107–120.

Louko LJ, 1995, 'Phonological Characteristics of Young Children who Stutter', *Topics in Language Disorders* 15, pp48–59.

Louko LJ, Edwards M & Conture E, 1990, 'Phonological Characteristics of Young Stutterers and their Normally Fluent Peers. Preliminary Observations', *Journal of Fluency Disorders* 15, pp191–210.

Manolson A, 1992, *It Takes 2 To Talk*, Hanen Centre, Ontario, Canada.

Mansson H, 2000, 'Childhood Stuttering: Incidence and Development', *Journal of Fluency Disorders* 25, pp47–57.

Matthews S, Williams R & Pring T, 1997, 'Parent-child Interaction Therapy and Dysfluency: A Single-case Study', *European Journal of Disorders of Communication* 32, pp346–357.

Melnick KS & Conture EG, 2000, 'Relationship of Length and Grammatical Complexity to the Systematic and Nonsystematic Speech Errors and Stuttering of Children who Stutter', *Journal of Fluency Disorders* 25, pp21–45.

Meyers SC & Freeman FJ, 1985a, 'Mother and Child Speech Rates as a Variable in Stuttering and Disfluency', *Journal of Speech and Hearing Research* 28, pp436–444.

Meyers SC & Freeman FJ, 1985b, 'Interruptions as a Variable in Stuttering and Disfluency', *Journal of Speech and Hearing Research* 28, pp428–435.

Meyers SC & Woodford LL, 1992, *The Fluency Development System for Young Children*, United Educational Services Inc, Buffalo, NY.

Miles S & Bernstein Ratner NB, 2001, 'Parental Language Input to Children at Stuttering Onset', *Journal of Speech, Language and Hearing Research* 44, pp1116–1130.

Millard SK, 2002, 'Therapy Outcome: Parents' Perspectives', Baker KL, Rustin L & Cook F (eds), *Proceedings of the Sixth Oxford Dysfluency Conference,* Kevin L Baker, Windsor.

Millard SK, Nicholas A & Cook FM, 2008, 'Is Parent-child Interaction Therapy Effective in Reducing Stuttering?' *Journal of Speech, Language and Hearing Research* 51(3), pp636–650.

Montgomery JW, 2005, 'Effects of Input Rate and Age on the Real-time Language Processing of Children with Specific Language Impairment', *International Journal of Language and Communication Disorders* 40, pp171–188.

Mordecai D, 1979, 'An Investigation of the Communicative Styles of Mothers and Fathers of Stuttering Versus Non-stuttering Pre-school Children', *Dissertations Abstracts International* 40, (4759B).

Nelson KE, Welsh J, Camarata SM, Butkovsky L & Camarata M, 1996, 'Effects of Conversational Recasting on the Acquisition of Grammar in Children with Specific Language Impairment and Younger Language-normal Children', *Journal of Speech and Hearing Research* 39, pp850–859.

Neumann K, Euler HA, von Gudenberg AW, Griraud AL, Lanfermann H & Gall V, 2000, 'The Nature and Treatment of Stuttering as Revealed by fMRI. A Within and Between Group Comparison', *Journal of Fluency Disorders* 28, pp381–410.

Newman LL & Smit AB, 1989, 'Some Effects of Variations in Response Time Latency on Speech Rate, Interruptions, and Fluency in Children's Speech', *Journal of Speech and Hearing Research* 32, pp635–644.

Nicholas A, Millard SK & Cook FM, 2004, 'Parent-child Interaction Therapy: Child and Parent Variables Pre and Post Therapy', Packmann A, Meltzer A & Peters HFM (eds), *Fluency Disorders: Theory, Research and Therapy in Fluency Disorders. Proceedings of the Fourth World Congress on Fluency Disorders*, University of Nijmegen Press, Nijmegen, The Netherlands.

Nicholas A, Yairi E, Davis S, Mangelsdorf S, Cook F & Hamilton V, 2006, 'A Study Investigating the Temperament of School-aged Children who Stutter', *Proceedings of the Fifth World Congress on Fluency Disorders, Dublin, Ireland, 25–28th July, 2006.*

Nippold MA, 1990, 'Concomitant Speech and Language Disorders in Stuttering Children: A Critique of the Literature', *Journal of Speech and Hearing Disorders* 55, pp51–60.

Nippold MA, 2002, 'Stuttering and Phonology: Is There an Interaction?' *American Journal of Speech-Language Pathology* 11, pp99–110.

Nippold MA, 2004, 'Phonological and Language Disorders in Children who Stutter: Impact on Treatment Recommendations', *Clinical Linguistics and Phonetics* 18, pp145–159.

Nippold MA & Rudzinski M, 1995, 'Parents' Speech and Children's Stuttering: A Critique of the Literature', *Journal of Speech and Hearing Research* 38, pp978–989.

O'Hanlon W & Weiner-Davis M, 1989, *In Search of Solutions*, Norton, New York, NY.

Onslow M, 2004, 'Treatment of Stuttering in Preschool Children', *Behaviour Change* 21, pp201–214.

Onslow M, Andrews C & Lincoln M, 1994, 'A Control/Experimental Trial of an Operant Treatment for Early Stuttering', *Journal of Speech and Hearing Research* 37, pp1244–1259.

Onslow M, Costa L & Rue S, 1990, 'Direct Early Intervention with Stuttering: Some Preliminary Data', *Journal of Speech and Hearing Disorders* 55, pp405–416.

Onslow M, Packman A & Harrison E, 2003, *The Lidcombe Program of Early Stuttering Intervention*, Pro-Ed, TX.

Oyler E & Ramig PR, 1995, 'Vulnerability in Stuttering Children', Session presented at the annual convention of the American Speech-Language-Hearing Association, Orlando, FL, December 1995.

Oyler ME, 1996, 'Vulnerability in Stuttering Children', *Dissertation Abstracts International: The Humanities and Social Sciences* 56, p3374.

Paden EP & Yairi E, 1996, 'Phonological Characteristics of Children whose Stuttering Persisted or Recovered', *Journal of Speech and Hearing Research* 39, pp981–990.

Paden EP, Yairi E & Ambrose NG, 1999, 'Early Childhood Stuttering II: Initial Status of Phonological Abilities', *Journal of Speech, Language and Hearing Research* 42, pp1113-1124.

Pellowski MW, Conture E, Anderson JD & Ohde RN, 2000, 'Articulatory and Phonological Assessment of Children who Stutter', Bosshardt HG, Yaruss JS & Peters HFM (eds), *Fluency Disorders: Theory, Research, Treatment and Self-help. Proceedings of the Third World Congress on Fluency Disorders,* University of Nijmegen Press, Nyborg, Denmark.

Peters H, Hulstijn W & Van Lieshout P, 2000, 'Recent Developments in Speech Motor Research and Stuttering', *Folia Phoniatrica et Logopaedica* 52, pp103–119.

Poulos MG & Webster WG, 1991, 'Family History as a Basis for Subgrouping People who Stutter', *Journal of Speech and Hearing Research* 34, pp5–10.

Pring T, 2004, 'Ask a Silly Question: Two Decades of Troublesome Trials', *International Journal of Language and Communication Disorders* 39, pp285–302.

Pring T, 2005, *Research Methods in Communication Disorders*, Whurr Publishers, London.

Ratner N & Silverman S, 2000, 'Parental Perceptions of Children's Communicative Development at Stuttering Onset', *Journal of Speech, Language and Hearing Research* 43, pp1252–1263.

Riley GD & Riley J, 1979, 'A Component Model for Diagnosing and Treating Children Who Stutter', *Journal of Fluency Disorders* 4, pp279–293.

Riley GD & Riley J, 1980, 'Motoric and Linguistic Variables among Children who Stutter: A Factor Analysis', *Journal of Speech and Hearing Disorders* 45, pp504–513.

Robey RR & Schultz MC, 1998, 'A Model for Conducting Clinical-outcome Research: An Adaptation for Use in Aphasiology', *Aphasiology* 12, pp787–810.

Rommel D, 2000, 'The Influence of Psycholinguistic Variables on Stuttering in Childhood', Bosshardt HG, Yaruss JS & Peters HFM (eds), *Fluency Disorders: Theory, Research, Treatment and Self-help. Proceedings of the Third World Congress on Fluency Disorders,* University of Nijmegen Press, Nyborg, Denmark.

Rommel D, Hage A, Kalehne P & Johannsen HS, 1999, 'Development, Maintenance and Recovery of Childhood Stuttering: Prospective Longitudinal Data 3 Years after First Contact', Baker KL, Rustin L & Cook F (eds), *Proceedings of the Fifth Oxford Dysfluency Conference,* Kevin L Baker, Oxford.

Runyan CM & Runyan SE, 1999, 'Therapy for School-aged Stutterers: An Update on the Fluency Rules Program', Curlee R (ed), *Stuttering and Related Disorders of Fluency,* pp101–123, Thieme, New York, NY.

Rustin L, 1987, *Assessment and Therapy Programme for Dysfluent Children*, NFER Nelson, Berkshire.

Rustin L & Cook F, 1995, 'Parental Involvement in the Treatment of Stuttering', *Language, Speech and Hearing Services in Schools* 26, pp127–137.

Rustin L, Botterill W & Kelman E, 1996, *Assessment and Therapy for Young Dysfluent Children: Family Interaction*, Whurr Publishers, London.

Ryan BP, 1992, 'Articulation, Language, Rate, and Fluency Characteristics of Stuttering and Nonstuttering Preschool Children', *Journal of Speech and Hearing Research* 35, pp333–342.

Schmidt U, 2005, 'Engagement and Motivational Interviewing', Graham P (ed), *Cognitive Behaviour Therapy for Children and Families*, Cambridge University Press, Cambridge.

Silverman EM, 1974, 'Word Position and Grammatical Function in Relation to Preschoolers' Speech Disfluency', *Perceptual and Motor Skills* 39, pp267–272.

Silverman S & Ratner NB, 2002, 'Measuring Lexical Diversity in Children who Stutter: Application of Vocd', *Journal of Fluency Disorders* 27, pp289–304.

Smith A & Kelly E, 1997, 'Stuttering: A Dynamic, Multifactorial Model', Curlee R & Siegel GM (eds), *Nature and Treatment of Stuttering: New Directions*, Allyn & Bacon, Boston, MA.

Smith CB, Adamson LB & Bakeman R, 1988, 'Interactional Predictors of Early Language', *First Language* 8, pp143–156.

Sommer M, Koch MA, Paulus W, Weiller C & Buchel C, 2002, 'Disconnection of Speech-relevant Brain Areas in Persistent Developmental Stuttering', *Lancet* 360, pp380–383.

Spinelli E, 1994, *Demistifying Therapy*, Constable, London.

Starkweather CW, 2002, 'The Epigenesis of Stuttering', *Journal of Fluency Disorders* 27, pp269–288.

Starkweather CW & Gottwald SR, 1990, 'The Demands and Capacities Model II: Clinical Applications', *Journal of Fluency Disorders* 15, pp143–157.

Starkweather CW, Gottwald SR & Halfond MM, 1990, *Stuttering Prevention: A Clinical Method*, Prentice-Hall, Englewood Cliffs, NJ.

Stephenson-Opsal D & Bernstein Ratner N, 1988, 'Maternal Speech Rate Modification and Childhood Stuttering', *Journal of Fluency Disorders* 15, pp243–175.

Stern E, 1948, 'A Preliminary Study of Bilingualism and Stuttering in Four Johannesburg Schools', *Journal of Logopaedics* 1, pp15–25.

Stewart S & Turnbull J, 2007, *Working with Dysfluent Children: Practical Approaches to Assessment and Therapy*, Speechmark, Milton Keynes.

Straus SE, Richardson WS, Glasziou P & Haynes RB, 2005, *Evidence-Based Medicine: How To Practice and Teach EBM*, Elsevier, Churchill Livingstone, London.

Tomasello M & Farrar MJ, 1986, 'Joint Attention and Early Language', *Child Development* 57, pp1454–1463.

Tomasello M & Todd J, 1983, 'Joint Attention and Lexical Acquisition Style', *First Language* 4, pp197–212.

Travis LE, Johnson W & Shrover J, 1937, 'The Relation of Bilingualism to Stuttering', *Journal of Speech Disorders* 2, pp185–189.

Van Borsel J, Maes E & Foulon S, 2001, 'Stuttering and Bilingualism: A Review', *Journal of Fluency Disorders* 26, pp179–205.

Vanryckeghem M & Brutten GJ, 1997, 'The Speech-associated Attitude of Children Who Do and Do Not Stutter and the Differential Effect of Age', *American Journal of Speech-Language Pathology* 6, pp67–73.

Vanryckeghem M, Brutten GJ & Hernandez LM, 2005, 'A Comparative Investigation of the Speech-associated Attitude of Preschool and Kindergarten Children who Do and Do Not Stutter', *Journal of Fluency Disorders* 30, pp307–318.

Wakaba Y, 1998, 'Research on Temperament of Stuttering Children with Early Onset', Paper presented at the Second World Congress on Fluency Disorders, San Francisco, CA, August, 1997.

Wall M & Myers F, 1995, *Clinical Management of Childhood Stuttering*, Pro-Ed, Austin, TX.

Wall MJ, Starkweather CW & Cairns HS, 1981, 'Syntactic Influences on Stuttering in Young Child Stutterers', *Journal of Fluency Disorders* 6, pp283–298.

Wampold BE, 2001, *The Great Psychotherapy Debate: Models, Methods and Findings*, Lawrence Erlbaum Associates, London.

Watkins K, Smith SM, Davis S & Howell P, 2007, 'Structural and Functional Abnormalities of the Motor System in Developmental Stuttering', *Brain*, pp1–10.

Watkins R, 2005, 'Language Abilities in Young Children who Stutter', Paper presented at the Sixth Oxford Dysfluency Conference, July 2005, Oxford.

Watkins RV & Johnson BW, 2004, 'Language Abilities in Children who Stutter: Toward Improved Research and Clinical Applications', *Language, Speech and Hearing Services in Schools* 35, pp82–89.

Watkins RV & Yairi E, 1997, 'Language Production Abilities of Children whose Stuttering Persisted or Recovered', *Journal of Speech, Language and Hearing Research* 40, pp385–399.

Watkins RV, Yairi E & Ambrose NG, 1999, 'Early Childhood Stuttering III: Initial Status of Expressive Language Abilities', *Journal of Speech, Language and Hearing Research* 42, pp1125–1135.

Weiss AL & Zebrowski PM, 1991, 'Patterns of Assertiveness and Responsiveness in Parental Interactions with Stuttering and Fluent Children', *Journal of Fluency Disorders* 16, pp125–141.

Weiss AL & Zebrowski PM, 1992, 'Disfluencies in the Conversations of Young Children who Stutter: Some Answers about Questions', *Journal of Speech and Hearing Research* 35, pp1230–1238.

Weiss A & Zebrowski PM, 2000, 'Adult-Child Conversation Contexts and Fluency: Who's Leading Whom?' Bosshardt HG, Yaruss JS & Peters HFM (eds), *Fluency Disorders: Theory, Research, Treatment and Self-help. Proceedings of the Third World Congress on Fluency Disorders,* University of Nijmegen Press, Nyborg, Denmark.

Weistuch L, Lewis M & Sullivan M, 1991, 'Use of a Language Interaction Intervention in the Preschools', *Journal of Early Intervention* 15, pp278–287.

Wilkenfeld JR & Curlee RF, 1997, 'The Relative Effects of Questions and Comments on Children's Stuttering', *American Journal of Speech-Language Pathology* 6, pp79–89.

Winslow M & Guitar B, 1994, 'The Effects of Structured Turn Taking on Disfluencies: A Case Study', *Language, Speech and Hearing Services in Schools* 25, pp251–257.

Wolk L, 1998, 'Intervention Strategies for Children who Exhibit Coexisting Phonological and Fluency Disorders: A Clinical Note', *Child Language Teaching and Therapy* 14, pp69–82.

Yairi E, 1983, 'The Onset of Stuttering in Two- and Three-year-old Children', *Journal of Speech and Hearing Disorders* 48, pp171–177.

Yairi E & Ambrose N, 1992a, 'A Longitudinal Study of Stuttering in Children: A Preliminary Report', *Journal of Speech and Hearing Research* 35, pp755–760.

Yairi E & Ambrose N, 1992b, 'Onset of Stuttering in Preschool Children: Selected Factors', *Journal of Speech and Hearing Research* 35, pp782–788.

Yairi E & Ambrose N, 1999, 'Early Childhood Stuttering I: Persistency and Recovery Rates', *Journal of Speech, Language and Hearing Research* 42, pp1097–1112.

Yairi E & Ambrose N, 2005, *Early Childhood Stuttering: For Clinicians, by Clinicians*, Pro-Ed, Austin, TX.

Yairi E, Ambrose NG & Niermann R, 1993, 'The Early Months of Stuttering: A Developmental Study', *Journal of Speech and Hearing Research* 36, pp521–528.

Yairi E, Ambrose NG, Paden EP & Throneburg RN, 1996, 'Predictive Factors of Persistence and Recovery: Pathways of Childhood Stuttering', *Journal of Communication Disorders* 29, pp51–77.

Yaruss JS, 1997, 'Clinical Implications of Situational Variability in Preschool Children who Stutter', *Journal of Fluency Disorders* 22, pp187–203.

Yaruss JS, 1999, 'Utterance Length, Syntactic Complexity, and Childhood Stuttering', *Journal of Speech, Language and Hearing Research* 42, pp329–344.

Yaruss JS & Conture EG, 1995, 'Mother and Child Speaking Rates and Utterance Lengths in Adjacent Fluent Utterances: Preliminary Observations', *Journal of Fluency Disorders* 20, pp257–278.

Yaruss JS, Coleman C & Hammer D, 2006, 'Treating Preschool Children who Stutter: Description and Preliminary Evaluation of a Family-focused Treatment Approach', *Language, Speech and Hearing Services in Schools* 37, pp118–136.

Yoder PJ & Warren SF, 1993, 'Can Developmentally Delayed Children's Language Development be Enhanced through Prelinguistic Intervention?' Kaiser AP & Gray SF (eds), *Enhancing Children's Communication: Research Foundations for Intervention*, pp35–61, Paul H. Brookes, Baltimore, MD.

Zackheim CT & Conture EG, 2003, 'Childhood Stuttering and Speech Disfluencies in Relation to Children's Mean Length of Utterance: A Preliminary Study', *Journal of Fluency Disorders* 28, pp115–141.

Zebrowski PM, 1995, 'Temporal Aspects of the Conversations between Children who Stutter and their Parents', *Topics in Language Disorders* 15, pp1–17.

Zebrowski PM & Schum RL, 1993, 'Counseling Parents of Children who Stutter', *American Journal of Speech-Language Pathology* 2, pp65–73.

Zebrowski PM, Weiss AL, Savelkoul EM & Hammer CS, 1996, 'The Effect of Maternal Rate Reduction on the Stuttering, Speech Rates and Linguistic Productions of Children who Stutter: Evidence from Individual Dyads', *Clinical Linguistics and Phonetics* 10, pp189–206.

Zenner AA, Ritterman SI, Bowen S & Gronhord KD, 1978, 'Measurement and Comparison of Anxiety Levels of Parents of Stuttering, Articulatory Defective and Non-stuttering Children', *Journal of Fluency Disorders* 3, pp273–283.

Index

G

H

I

L

M

N

O

P

T

V

W